# The
# Compassionate
# Carnivore

## Also by Catherine Friend

NONFICTION:
*Hit by a Farm: How I Learned to
Stop Worrying and Love the Barn*

NOVELS:
*The Spanish Pearl*
*The Crown of Valencia*

CHILDREN'S:
*The Perfect Nest*
*Eddie the Racoon*
*Silly Ruby*

# The
# Compassionate
# Carnivore

Or, How to Keep Animals Happy,
Save Old MacDonald's Farm,
Reduce Your Hoofprint,
and Still Eat Meat

## *Catherine Friend*

Da Capo
LIFE
LONG

A Member of the Perseus Books Group

Designed by Pauline Brown
Set in 11.5 point Garamond by the Perseus Books Group

Library of Congress Cataloging-in-Publication Data

Friend, Catherine.
   The compassionate carnivore : or, how to keep animals happy, save Old Macdonald's Farm, reduce your hoofprint, and still eat meat / Catherine Friend.
      p. cm.
   Includes bibliographical references and index.
   ISBN 978-1-60094-007-1 (hardcover : alk. paper)
   1. Meat. 2. Consumers—Attitudes. 3. Meat animals. 4. Animal welfare. I. Title. II. Title: How to keep animals happy, save Old Macdonald's Farm, reduce your hoofprint, and still eat meat.
   TX371.F74 2008
   641.3'6—dc22

                                            2007043979

First Da Capo Press edition 2008

Published by Da Capo Press
A Member of the Perseus Books Group
www.dacapopress.com

Da Capo Press books are available at special discounts for bulk purchases in the United States by corporations, institutions, and other organizations. For more information, please contact the Special Markets Department at the Perseus Books Group, 2300 Chestnut Street, Suite 200, Philadelphia, PA 19103, or call (800) 255-1514, or e-mail special. markets@perseusbooks.com.

1 2 3 4 5 6 7 8 9

*To the farmers
who raise animals humanely
and the consumers who seek them out*

# Contents

••• ••• •••••• ••• •••

Part One

# What's a
# Carnivore to Do?

Just as boats of various designs leave very different
wakes in the water behind them, so too do various
approaches to living send out different waves of
reverberating influence on the world.

—DUANE ELGIN

L ife as a carnivore used to be simple. Our choices were straightforward: Original Recipe or Extra Crispy? Pork ribs or beef ribs? Chicken pot pie or turkey pot pie? Today, however, in the brave new world of increased awareness of environmental impact, health concerns, and animal welfare, the choices are no longer just between specific *dishes,* but between different ways to raise, feed, and butcher the animals that become the meat *in* those dishes. The choices are so dizzying that, to paraphrase Dr. Emilio Lazardo in *The Adventures of Buckaroo Bonzai,* it's enough to make the ganglia twitch.

At the grocery store, do I pay ninety-nine cents for the regular eggs, or four dollars for the cage-free eggs? How can I eat out if I can't find a restaurant that serves meat raised the way I want it raised? Do I spend time finding farmers who raise meat animals humanely, or do I close my eyes and buy the stuff at the store that's been raised in a factory because I don't have time to look for anything else? Should I buy grass-fed or grass-finished meat? Corn-fed? Pasture-raised or feedlot-raised? No antibiotics? No growth hormones? Do I buy organic meat shipped one thousand miles, or nonorganic meat shipped sixty miles? Should I buy meat from a small but conventional farm? Heck, should I even be eating meat at all?

Unfortunately, I don't believe there are clear answers to any of these questions. For example, researchers have found that most of the food we eat has traveled at least fifteen hundred miles before it reaches our plate, and because that transportation consumes a great deal of fossil fuel and emits plenty of carbon dioxide, the conclusion is that we should all eat locally. But an op-ed piece in the *New York Times* raised the opposite idea. New Zealand researchers now claim that the process of raising lamb on a clover-rich New Zealand pasture and shipping it eleven thousand miles to Great Britain emits much less carbon dioxide than the process of raising a lamb on grain in England itself.[1]

I can feel my ganglia starting to twitch already. On my cynical days I wonder if there are any truths I can trust about becoming a more compassionate carnivore.

On my less cynical days, I know there are. As I waded through what it means to be a carnivore today, I kept coming back to the one thing that *I* know to be true: the animals themselves matter. Treating animals with respect and consideration is an act that sends out ever-widening ripples into the world. To begin down this path, all we need to do is pull our heads up out of the sand.

# Pulling My Head
# Out of the Sand

... ... ...... ... ...

FOR ME, IT'S all about the animals, because I am a farmer and I raise animals for meat. I wasn't raised on a farm and had no dreams of farming, but in the mid-1990s, my partner, Melissa, confessed she'd always wanted to be a farmer and asked if I would help her start a farm.

What happened when I said yes is a long story, but the short version is that today we run a small sustainable farm and raise sheep. We have three guard llamas for protecting the flock, and we sometimes have goats. We sell lamb, duck, and chicken eggs. Melissa is in her element, repairing the tractor, fixing fences, and taking care of the animals. I tend to resist getting my hands dirty (an endearing phobia that apparently began when I was a toddler and refused to finger-paint), but I provide valuable backup when the sheep get out (and chaos ensues), and I help with the farm's management and planning. Over the last fifteen years my perspective has shifted from city to rural, from consumer to producer, from livestock-ignorant to livestock-familiar. I am fiercely proud of the farm we've created and how we raise our animals.

Until Melissa and I started our farm, I'd lived in the city, where I happily wore clean clothes, kept a tidy house, paid no attention to the changing seasons, and was content to completely ignore the fact that my meat used to be an animal's muscles. While ostriches don't really stick their heads in the sand to hide (they stretch out flat against the ground), the whole head-in-the-sand thing beautifully described my approach to eating meat. Meat came from Styrofoam trays covered in cellophane, all traces of skin and blood and guts removed, so I could easily forget that the meat used to be an animal. I didn't want to know that Bessie in the barn had become the burger on my bun.

But now I do know. And as I've learned more about farming, and about eating meat, and about raising animals humanely, I've learned there is no right way to become a more compassionate carnivore. I love meat and am not going to give it up. There'll be no 100-mile or 250-mile local diet for this chick, although I commend those who are willing to take on the challenge. No feeding myself entirely from my garden, which I do not have and do not intend to plant, because, truth be told, I'm not all that wild about vegetables, only eating them because my mother tells me I must. I don't enjoy cooking. As comedian Carrie Snow said: "I prefer Hostess fruit pies to pop-up toaster tarts, because they don't require as much cooking."

Because of my concern for the environment, the lives of animals, and my own health, I've spent the last ten years exploring how to make better choices in the meat I buy. Hopefully my experiences will help you bridge the yawning gap between the ideal and the real, since our realistic choices may be very different from our philosophical choices. This book is not a declaration of war against farmers, since I am one. It's not a plea for everyone to become a vegetarian, since I will never be one.

This will not be one of those cheerful self-help books that makes change sound so ridiculously *easy*—"Become a Compassionate

Carnivore in Just Ten Days!"—that you feel like a total loser when you're not able to pull it off. At the other extreme, it's not intended to be one of those books about factory farming that's so depressing that you can't get out of bed for a week. There's only one rule you need to keep in mind as you approach the idea of becoming a more conscientious, compassionate carnivore, and here it is: the first being on whom you must practice compassion is yourself.

So what's a compassionate carnivore to do when faced with new choices and conflicting information? We can learn more about our choices, then decide what's important for us and for our families. Scattered throughout the book are ideas for steps you can take, and when I've herded them all together at the end, you'll have a good range of choices from which to select.

Here's a heads-up, though: becoming a more compassionate carnivore requires change, and change requires time, the one thing most of us lack. How can we possibly change *how* we eat when we barely have enough time *to* eat?

Carl Honoré said this about today's fast pace of life: "The more everyone else bangs on about how fast the world is, the more we assume that slowing down is impossible." Yet by the end of his book *In Praise of Slowness,* we learn that slowing down isn't impossible: "The Slow philosophy delivers the things that really make us happy: good health, a thriving environment, strong communities and relationships, freedom from perpetual hurry."[2] I'm hoping that by the end of this book, you'll want to slow down a bit. You'll want to pay more attention to where your meat comes from and how it was raised.

Most of us have distanced ourselves from our meat, protecting ourselves from the truth that we are eating animals. Yet we don't need to protect ourselves. Ignorance is not bliss. Being a carnivore who's asleep at the wheel means someone else is driving. Being a carnivore who wakes up, looks around, and engages means you're in charge. Being in charge is good.

So in this book I'll explore some of the basic issues—why it might be hard to change how we eat meat, and what it means to pay more attention to the animals we eat. Next will be a brief look at our current meat-eating habits, and whether that's a good place in which to be.

There's no avoiding a discussion of some of the nasty effects of factory farming, both on animals and the environment, and some of you will feel so guilty you'll put the book down and be done with the whole thing. Enough with the guilt. I've struggled with it for years and have finally accepted that it's a total waste of time. Instead of giving in to guilt, resolve to stay awake and accept that you can do nothing about what's happened up to this point. We start from here, from today.

I'll discuss sustainable and organic alternatives to factory meat, and how what an animal is fed will affect meat taste and quality. I'll cover what we all want to avoid, and that's the process of how animals become meat. For a break, I'll take you on a relaxing pasture walk, then we'll get creative about finding sources for the kind of meat you want to buy.

This is an exciting time to be both a carnivore and a farmer, and I'm optimistic we're approaching a tipping point when it comes to buying meat from animals raised humanely. Of course, I might just be the optimist Gretel Erhlich once described, the guy who fell off a ten-story building, and as he passed each floor, said, "Well, I'm all right so far."

Let's hope not.

Farmers and consumers have finally found each other. Thanks to farmers markets, the Internet, and other methods, you and I can connect more easily than ever before. We can support one another by totally bypassing today's food distribution system, and in doing so, I'm positive we can create better lives for meat animals, farmers, and consumers alike.

# Pork-Chop-
# on-a-Stick

··· ··· ······ ··· ···

THE ONLY TIME I really connected the food on my plate with an animal in the barn was as a child, when my sheep-raising Montana grandmother came to visit and cooked a beef dish so tasty that my sister and I had a fork fight over the last piece. Turned out Grandma, whom I *thought* had loved us, had fed us beef tongue. I had a tongue. A cow had a tongue, and I'd just eaten it. Lordy. That was enough reality for this girl, so I quickly built a nice tall wall around the truth, and life was once again good.

But then Melissa and I took the plunge into farming and that wall came tumbling down. The sheep and chickens knocked it over. Suddenly not only was I surrounded by animals, but they were animals whose only reason for being there was to be killed and eaten. I met my meat, looked it in the eye, patted it on the head, and even kissed it on the nose now and then. (Not chickens, however. I had standards.) I could no longer ignore the fact that my food had a face.

During those first few years as a farmer, my carnivorous consciousness sprang to life. I liked the idea of raising meat animals humanely on a small farm. Farm animals should have good lives, I believed, even if they didn't live all that long. In fact, the motto for our animals' lives became "quality, not quantity."

We moved the sheep to fresh pasture every day so that they could harvest the grass and distribute their own manure. We raised the chickens in moveable pens that kept them safe from predators but allowed them to graze and eat bugs. Within a year, tucked away in our big freezer we had lamb, which we'd raised, and chicken, which we'd raised. I bought some pork from a guy named Dennis who let his hogs graze outside, and I was set.

Over the next few years, working on the farm consumed my life as we built buildings, put up fences, ran water lines throughout the pasture, and mowed. Because I had little energy for cooking, I stopped paying attention to *what* I was cooking. While we still ate our own lamb, we stopped raising chickens, because we were losing money at it and found moving the pens exhausting. I started buying chicken from the grocery store again. When we ran out of Dennis's pork, I never seemed to find the time to call him and order more, so I started buying pork from the grocery store again. I never considered the environmental implications of my purchases nor the impact on animals' lives or my own. Without intending to, I'd built up that wall again. I'd stuck my ostrich head back into the sand. But then I went to the Minnesota State Fair and got knocked flat on my faux–compassionate carnivore butt.

The Minnesota State Fair, which can best be described as a food orgy, is known for its food on a stick—cheeseburger-on-a-stick, Bananas-Foster-on-a-stick, Puff-Daddy-on-a-stick (spiced sausage), deep-fried-cheesecake-on-a-stick, mocha-on-a-stick. If a stick can be stuck into a food, someone has done so at the Minnesota State Fair. Fried foods are another favorite—deep-fried candy bars, deep-fried fruit, deep-fried Spam cubes.

The state fair is also a huge party that celebrates agriculture. There's the cooled booth where a sculptor carves ninety-pound blocks of butter into the likenesses of each of the Princess Kay of the Milky Way candidates, young women competing to be the goodwill ambassador for the Minnesota dairy industry. The candidates wear thick parkas to stay warm as they model.

There's the crop art, where artists use thousands of crop seeds to create likenesses of everyone from Elvis, to Lucy and Desi, to the Pope, to Garrison Keillor. The artists are amazing, actually.

And although the fair has shifted its focus enough from rural to urban that Machinery Hill is gone—not many city dwellers are interested in combines or balers—the agricultural attraction that remains is the animals. At the west end of the fairgrounds you'll find huge concrete buildings for cattle, swine, poultry, sheep, and goats. In the cattle building there are beef and dairy animals bedded down on thick pads of straw. Teenage FFA and 4-H members scoop up manure, wash their cows, sit in bunches and talk, or stretch out next to their cows and grab some sleep. It's a jaw-dropping sight to see a one-hundred-pound teenage girl curled up back-to-back with her fifteen-hundred-pound Holstein cow, the girl sound asleep, the cow calmly chewing its cud.

As I walked through the animal barns, seeing goats, sheep, swine, poultry, and llamas, I was struck by what an amazing opportunity this was for city kids. I passed a young boy sitting on his haunches, gazing through the pen bars into the eyes of a Toggenburg dairy goat. Outside another pen, young fingers reached for their first feel of wool. Unless kids get out of the city and visit farms such as ours, the state fair is one of the few places where urban children have the opportunity to see and touch living, breathing farm animals.

One of the most popular buildings the last few years has been the Miracle of Birth barn—a crowded spot where fairgoers can watch pregnant ewes, sows, and cows give birth. If the crowds were too great to get close to the birth in progress, large TV screens overhead shared the births. Newborn lambs slept in one pen. A wobbly-legged calf stood next to Mama in another. The crowd was thick around a farrowing pen, and I looked up at the TV just in time to see a tiny piglet come squirting out. The crowd oohed and aahed.

The cozy "Mama and baby in the straw" scenes in the newly remodeled and updated Miracle of Birth barn touched everyone's hearts. But that day at the fair, when the crowd around the piglets parted, I could neither understand nor believe what I saw.

Stretched out on her side in a raised pen was a massive white sow, her two rows of swollen teats exposed so that the piglets could easily feed. Days-old piglets either slept in piles alongside the sow or nursed energetically. I wondered why the sow was so still. She must have been sleeping. Then I realized there were three more pens just like this one, and none of the sows were moving, not a twitch. Good lord, were they dead?

I kept changing position, trying to see through the crowds. The blue bars of the pen were attractive and clean and new. They seemed so narrow. Could the sow even stand up? How could she possibly interact with and nuzzle her babies? Her head was barely visible, so close to the silver metal panel by her head that I couldn't see her face.

It hit me in the gut. For the first time I was seeing what I'd only vaguely heard about—the industrial practice of raising pigs. Instead of letting the sow live naturally, agriculture had turned her into nothing more than a milk machine for piglets. As people pushed past me to get a closer look at the piglets, my eyes flickered to the sign overhead, which proudly proclaimed that vets had developed this pen to ensure that sows wouldn't lie down and crush their own piglets, and that the sows were kept in these pens for twenty-one days.

Talk about blaming the victim. A sow's natural behavior is to build a nest of straw or sticks, give birth, and tend her babies. When given adequate room in which to do this, sows know perfectly well where their babies are and don't squash them. However, when industrial agriculture put sows in pens so narrow they couldn't turn around, sows, sadly, crushed their babies. Yet this sign over my head implied that it was necessary for the sow to be restrained for three weeks because it was her natural behavior to sit on her babies.

I rushed over to one of the attendants in blue polo shirts to confront her, but she was busy, and I was too upset to speak anyway. I rushed back to the nearest farrowing pen, literally shaking with anger. The sows didn't even look like animals. They looked like long, white milk bladders. That not one of them even twitched struck me as unnatural. How could they lie there all day and not move?

The crowd adored the piglets. "Aren't they cute?" "Look at their little tails." "That one's hungry." I didn't know which was more upsetting: that the sows' restraints were presented as perfectly natural, or that no one else around me seemed to have noticed.

I ended up leaving without speaking to any of the attendants, so I would have to wait until next year to ask my questions. But my resolve to no longer support this sort of agricultural practice had been reignited. Instead, I would seek out other farmers who raised pork more naturally, who gave them bedding material and the room to make nests, who let them give birth and care for their piglets. I would become Super-Compassionate Carnivore, able to leap over inhumanely raised meat in a single bound.

After we left the Miracle of Birth barn in the early afternoon, we pressed on, visiting the shops beneath the grandstand, eating an elephant ear (a flat round pastry slathered in melted butter and powdered sugar), key-lime-pie-on-a-stick, fried cheese curds, garlic french fries, Tom Thumb mini doughnuts, freshly pulled saltwater taffy, and just watching the thousands of people milling about.

By 7:00 P.M. my feet ached, my back burned, I'd had it with the crowds, and it was time to go home. Quick—what last treats could we squeeze in before we left? Melissa loves the malts in the Empire Commons, which had a line as long as the Mississippi snaking through it, so she headed for the line, and I headed for my absolute favorite food on a stick.

Halfway down the block from the Empire Commons sat the pork-chop-on-a-stick booth. The pork chop is marinated in a great blend of spices, grilled to perfection, then jammed onto a stick. I waited in line patiently, knowing it would be worth the wait. Armed with my pork-chop-on-a-stick, a drink, and a handful of napkins, I headed back to our meeting place, found a bare square of grass, sat down, and ate every last bit of that pork chop, leaving only the bone. I think I might have actually sucked on that, too, my eyes closed in gluttonous bliss.

Not until I was halfway home did I realize what I had done. That pork chop had come from a pig raised in a factory.

Damn it.

# Can a Carnivore
# Be Compassionate?

••• ••• •••••• ••• •••

HUMANS ARE OMNIVORES, meaning we eat both plants and animals. Not to be insensitive to the lives of carrots, but I'm just not that concerned with the plant part of my diet. I don't feel guilty eating a carrot. What concerns me is the meat, or animal, part of my diet, which is why I use the word *carnivore* to describe myself. I also just like the word better because it gives me a bit of a jolt. It brings to mind lions and tigers and alligators. We humans aren't the only carnivores on the planet; we're just the ones who use forks or chopsticks.

When I mentioned the phrase "compassionate carnivore" to an outspoken vegetarian acquaintance of mine, she snorted and said, "Now *there's* an oxymoron." In her world, the only way to show compassion for an animal is not to eat it. If that's the only definition of *compassionate* allowed, then the discussion ends and nothing changes.

But in my world, a mixed bag of farm economics and loving animals and loving meat, I believe it's possible to show compassion for animals yet still eat them. For me, this means paying attention. It means learning more about the animals I eat and taking some responsibility for their quality of life. It means becoming a more aware, more *awake* carnivore who tries to alter her meat purchases to support her personal philosophies.

That said, as my pork-chop-on-a-stick debacle illustrates, I often fail miserably to do any of the above. What is wrong with me?

As an adult, I'm worried about tsunami victims and poverty in Africa and those people in New Orleans who still don't have any libraries. The polar ice caps are melting, so I must cut my fossil fuel use even more than I already have. The environment is constantly under attack, so I do my best to reduce, reuse, recycle. Politics is such a mess that sometimes I wonder if anything I do, including vote, will make any difference whatsoever. I haven't had my daily servings of fruits and vegetables for weeks, and I desperately wish there was a company that could inject all of my daily nutritional requirements into a bag of Cheetos. And that's on a good day.

Perhaps that's why making better choices in how I eat meat— how much, and from where—is so difficult for me. I'm overworked, overwhelmed, and, if truth be told, a tad lazy. If something's too hard, or takes too much time, I'm likely to give up. My path to becoming a compassionate carnivore has been paved with good intentions, but littered with the bones of pork-chop-on-a-stick.

After my state fair screw-up, I tried to figure out why change was such a challenge for me, and at first had more questions than answers. What did I need to become a more compassionate carnivore? What were the pitfalls to avoid? If I really paid more attention to meat animals—how they're raised, their habits, their emotional lives—could I still eat them? Would my food choices help animals, since they'd already been killed for meat?

I wish there were a neat and tidy way to corral each of these issues into its own chapter, but as fat runs through meat, these issues are marbled throughout the entire experience of eating meat. Making better choices, facing where our meat comes from, and understanding the impact of our purchases are all fibers of the same muscle.

I have learned that animal lovers who want to pay more attention to how meat animals are raised face two obstacles. The first is our tendency to view animals as a faceless group. Until I started farming, I honestly hadn't known that livestock animals had individual personalities, and that they had definite likes and dislikes. I tended to lump animals all together and rely on the anonymity that comes from talking about "sheep" and "beef cattle" and "hogs." It's hard to care about some faceless group of cattle or hogs. But as Jonathan Balcombe writes in *Pleasurable Kingdom,* "pleasures and pains are felt by individuals, not populations."[3]

As I became more comfortable with myself as a farmer, I began seeing animals as individuals, and therefore started caring deeply about the well-being of each of them. "Cattle" was an anonymous group, but "cow" had a face. Lamb #203 was a playful guy; #279 ran away if I even looked at him. Ewe #85 learned to jump fences and taught her twin lambs to do the same. We have a white hen who knows there are sunflower seeds in the shed, so whenever I head for the shed, she's right behind me, insistently stalking me until I give in and sprinkle some seeds on the ground.

A flock of sheep might contain one ewe who's cranky, one that'll do anything for a grain of corn, and another with wool dreadlocks dangling provocatively in her eyes. Living and working on a small farm forces me to see animals as individuals. There's no running away from the truth, no sticking my cute little ostrich head back into the sand. I now know that every piece of meat I eat comes from an animal with an ear tag number, a face, a history, a personality, a life. But when I race through the grocery store, already late for a meeting, or plan a day's meals when I'm facing a writing deadline, it can be very difficult to re-member that meat used to be an animal and to buy accordingly. A 2004 Ohio State University survey found that 81 percent of re-spondents felt that the well-being of livestock is as important as that of pets.[4] If that's true, why do so few people actually pay *at-tention* to this well-being?

The answer might be found in the second obstacle to being more compassionate, which is compassion itself. It turns out there is a limit to human compassion, which makes me uncomfortable. Journalist Nicholas Kristof wrote about a phenomenon psycholo-gists have discovered: that good, conscientious people often aren't moved by genocide or famines.[5] The idea of so many people in distress is hard for humans to get their minds around, so the hor-rible events fail to spark emotions that would lead to action. Samantha Power, author of *A Problem from Hell: America and the Age of Genocide,* says that when this happens, bystanders to geno-cides or other large disasters are able to "retreat to the 'twilight be-tween knowing and not knowing.'"[6] A sort of numbing results from our inability to appreciate losses as they become larger.

Research scientist Paul Slovic wrote: "Confronted with knowl-edge of dozens of apparently random disasters each day, what can a human heart do but slam its doors? No mortal can grieve that much. We didn't evolve to cope with tragedy on a global scale. Our defense is to pretend there's no thread of event that connects us, and that those lives are somehow not precious and real like our own. It's a practical strategy . . . but the loss of empathy is also the loss of humanity, and that's no small tradeoff."[7]

Studies show that people tend to react more strongly to the dis-tress of one individual: people would contribute more money to one child in Mali than to 21 million starving Africans. The same is true of animals. After a severe outbreak of foot-and-mouth dis-ease in Great Britain, standard policy was to destroy all the healthy animals within a certain distance from the diseased animals. As a result, millions of animals were slaughtered—600,000 cattle, 3.2 million sheep, and thousands of pigs, goats, and other animals—and they continued to be slaughtered even as the disease waned.[8]

Yet the plight of one animal touched the public more than the plight of all the thousands already killed. Just after a white calf had been born in Devon, England, an outbreak of foot-and-mouth disease on a neighboring farm required that all the animals on the calf's farm be killed, even if healthy. Employees of the Ministry of Agriculture showed up and administered lethal injections to fifteen cows and thirty sheep, then closed the doors of the barn. Five days later more ministry employees returned to disinfect the carcasses. They opened up the barn to find the white calf very much alive, standing next to its dead mother.

The farmers, delighted the animal was alive but horrified they hadn't known this so that they could have cared for it, quickly fed the animal, named her Phoenix, and called the press. The ministry still insisted the white calf be killed. But as the story circulated, public outcry was deafening, and the slaughter policy was quickly changed so that healthy animals on neighboring farms would no longer automatically be killed.[9]

I don't consider the deaths of livestock animals tragedies like famines or earthquakes or violent civil wars, because these animals are being raised for the purpose of feeding us. But because factory farms have grown so large and have become the predominant source of meat in this country, to think about the millions of animals living in this system every day creates, in me, such emotional numbing I find it almost impossible to care.

The irony, of course, is that most of us care deeply about wildlife animals. We care about the lives of wolves and deer and spotted owls and African elephants and panda bears. For some reason, Mother Nature in her wild state is noble and to be protected, but when it comes to Mother Nature's creatures that we enjoy eating, we have looked away.

As a result of looking away, I have allowed myself to become a baby barn swallow.

Barn swallows are considered good luck, so we happily let them build their mud nests in the rafters of our small barn. Every spring five or six baby birds peek over the sides of the nest to watch us work, looking clownish with their impossibly wide beaks and goofy tufts of feathers sticking up like baby Mohawks.

We watch when the babies are being fed. It's both hilarious and a little gross. The baby chirps impatiently until a parent returns to the nest, then the baby throws back its head, opens its mouth wide, and lets the parent stuff it full of regurgitated food, food that has been, well, processed.

When it comes to my food, meat or otherwise, for most of my life I've been a baby bird, tossing my head back, opening wide, and letting corporate agriculture—Cargill and ADM (Archer Daniels Midland) and ConAgra—feed me whatever they want. The baby bird doesn't know what Papa Bird is jamming down its throat, and it doesn't care. It just wants to be fed and will accept any level of processing for the convenience. Because I've paid corporations to feed me, I've sent the constant signal that whatever they put in the food and however they raise the animals is okay with me.

It's not okay anymore. Becoming a farmer has ruined my ability to ignore the impact modern agriculture has on animals, the environment, and me. I can no longer just throw back my head and let Papa Bird feed me.

In the 1930s and 1940s my grandmother on her Montana sheep ranch waited until the temperatures dropped below freezing in the fall and then butchered a sheep, gutted it, skinned it, and hung it out in the shed for the winter. Whenever she needed meat, she trudged out through the snow with a meat cleaver, hacked off enough frozen meat to feed her husband and three daughters, then, huddled against the bitter cold, returned to the house. I think of this whenever I resent standing in line at the grocery store.

To resist the whole Papa Bird thing, to change how I eat, means to take more responsibility for feeding myself. It doesn't mean I want to return to my grandmother's life. It doesn't mean I want to raise all of my own food. It just means I'm going to open my eyes and be more critical of what Papa Bird is stuffing in my mouth, and where it came from.

That's probably the first step anyone can take toward eating meat: pay more attention. To what? To everything: farms—how they work and don't work, and farm animals—how they live and how they die.

# I Learn a
# Few F-Words

••• ••• •••••• ••• •••

IT WAS HARD for me to learn more about farming without feeling a little bit stupid. When Melissa and I started our farm, I struggled to learn the differences between the types of farms. Were factory farms really farms? What the heck was a farm supposed to look like? Our farm doesn't have a big red barn; our buildings are tan metal with green metal roofs. Our farm doesn't have a quaint farmhouse reassuringly decorated with geese or rooster art. Instead, we live in a cedar-sided, fourteen-year-old house that has developed cracks in the drywall, dings in the doors, and the carpeting has lost that "just laid" look. (Hmmm, haven't we all. . . .)

I needed to learn more about farming without exposing my city-girl ignorance to other farmers, a tricky business. Take, for instance, the time I was mingling at a meeting of mostly male farmers who were wearing seed caps and overalls. I was actively pretending I belonged when a guy started talking to me about sheep. Since Melissa and I had just purchased a flock of fifty sheep, I figured I could easily talk sheep.

"So, you got any fat lambs?" the guy asked.

As a woman with curves, I was a bit sensitive to this F-word, but the guy wasn't laughing. The fact that he was deadly serious meant I didn't have a clue as to what "fat lamb" meant, and since Melissa wasn't nearby I had no choice but to jam my hands into my jean pockets and say, "Sure, doesn't everyone?"

The guy nodded, satisfied, and kept going. "I hear you lamb on pasture. Does that mean you also finish on grass?"

Finish? Did he mean finish as in "finish them off," killing the animals on the lawn instead of on the driveway? I jammed my hands deeper into those pockets and in a panic scanned the room for Melissa again, but she was too far away to help. "Sure, doesn't everyone?" I finally said.

The guy's eyebrow shot up. "Hardly anyone does," he said, and I made a mental note to find out what "finish" meant.

On my path to becoming a farmer, I had to learn more about animals—how to care for them, how to feed them, and how to make sure they're given what they need to lead what I would call a normal, natural life. What diseases could they get living in a barn? What diseases could they get living outside a barn? Why did farmers drench sheep and worm cattle and dust chickens? When were antibiotics good, and when were they bad?

I had to learn more about meat and the language that surrounds it. The first time we took a lamb into the butcher's, the butcher called the next day to get cutting instructions. I was stunned—he was asking *me* how to cut up the lamb carcass? Wasn't that his job? He rattled off a bunch of questions using mostly words I didn't recognize, or words in combinations I'd never heard before, like "Do you want the sirloin rolled with the roast?" I clenched my teeth, and in a panic once again scanned for Melissa, but she was outside doing chores. "Sure, doesn't everyone?" I finally said.

I eventually learned that to finish an animal means to raise it to market weight, the weight at which it is butchered. When some farmers refer to fat lambs or fat steers, they are talking about animals that have been fattened up to their market weight. An animal may spend its entire life on one farm. For example, some hog farms are farrow to finish, meaning the pigs are farrowed (born), then finished on the farm. Other farmers may buy animals that have been born on another farm and finish them.

How an animal has been finished will be a key factor in some of the decisions you'll make, since what the animal eats affects the taste of the meat. A farmer can finish an animal on grain, on grass, or on some combination of the two.

As we continued to build our farm, I ran smack up against another F-word: feedlot. Feedlot was a farming practice to be avoided at all costs. We were pasture-based. We were sustainable. No feedlots on this responsible little farm, since a feedlot is a fenced-in area where cattle or sheep or hogs stand around waiting to be fed. The grass is gone because the animals have trampled it or eaten it. On dry days they are standing around or lying down on dirt and manure. On wet days they are standing around or lying down in mud and manure. I've seen cattle up to their knees in something black and wet, and I know it wasn't just mud.

Then a few years into our farming career, Melissa informed me she was heading up to the county office to register our feedlot.

"Register our *what?*"

Melissa explained that the area where we winter our sheep is technically a feedlot, and since regulations had recently changed, she had to register the feedlot with the county. In the late fall the grass stops growing on our farm, so the food's gone. We bring the animals in closer to the barn and set up big round bales of hay, each weighing about eight hundred pounds, for them to eat. Before they start on the bales, however, animals will graze the vegetation down to nothing, and that's what creates a feedlot—bare soil. There is no vegetation to stop wind or water erosion, or to absorb the nutrients from the manure.

However, we make sure the area is large enough that there is still vegetation on the ground, that the animals aren't standing in manure, and that they have plenty of room to spread out if they want. Although there are muddy trails in the spring, the sheep have plenty of room to find dry ground, and their manure isn't that heavily concentrated.

I should also mention that many farmers who graze animals might call their feedlot a "sacrifice lot." I didn't realize how deeply I'd absorbed the jargon I was learning as a farmer until I took some friends on a tour of our relatively new farm and pointed out the sacrifice lot. They grew very quiet, and then one of them asked, "What do you sacrifice here?" They thought I meant sacrifice as in putting an animal on an altar and killing it. When you bring animals in from the pasture and set up hay bales for them to eat, the grass around those bales becomes overgrazed, trampled upon, and often doesn't grow back the next year. A farmer is sacrificing *grass*, not animals.

I was incensed to think a sustainable farm could have a feedlot. "Absolutely not," I sputtered at Melissa. "We are not calling that area a feedlot." Melissa gave me one of those "here we go again" looks, and since she prefers to follow rules and I prefer to break them, she registered our feedlot.

It turns out that most farms, especially northern farms, have feedlots and must be inspected to make sure concentrated manure isn't draining into a nearby watershed. I know now that feedlot isn't necessarily always a bad word, but is a reality on many farms. It's when those feedlots grow too large that problems begin.

It's difficult for me to remember that not everyone wants to know everything I know about farming, which is why it's hard for me not to share fascinating facts such as that feeding kelp to sheep keeps them healthy or that ducks have curly penises. So for now I'll stick to just finish and feedlot, because you'll need these concepts when you begin exploring different sources for meat. By the time you're through with this book, you'll be able to impress a room full of farmers with your knowledge of farming jargon, which I'm sure is everyone's secret desire.

# Meet Fluffy—
# She'll Be Your
# Lamb Chop Tonight

••• ••• •••••• ••• •••

I AM A FARMER and a carnivore, and some days neither rests easily on my shoulders. I've always assumed that farmers were totally comfortable with the idea of raising animals and then killing them for meat, yet for me, as a relatively new farmer, it's difficult to load up our animals and drive them to the butcher. We've been doing this for more than ten years now, and even though it certainly has become a normal part of my life, the act of paying someone to kill our animals never ceases to briefly—and sharply—take my breath away.

When Melissa and I started hanging around other farmers in southeastern Minnesota as newbie shepherds, one question formed in my head but never made it out of my lips: "Is it hard for you to have your animals killed and turned into meat?" To this day, I've never asked that question.

Farmers talk about the weather and its impact on crops or pasture regrowth. We talk about the high prices we pay for corn and the low prices we receive for wool and meat. We talk about fencing woes and fatal sheep diseases and vet bills. We don't talk about how it feels to raise an animal, have it killed, and then eat it.

I suppose that's because most farmers around here were raised on farms where killing and eating the animals they raised was such a natural part of life that it makes no sense to discuss it, sort of like discussing why grass is green or why the sun rises in the east. But for me the whole thing was mind-bogglingly intense.

Take the first time we gathered up our chickens for butchering the next day. Sixty chickens were living in a moveable, two-foot-high pen, so to reach them we removed part of the pen's lid and then Melissa crawled inside, slipping on the wet manure and mud. On her hands and knees, she caught each bird and handed it, flapping and squawking, up to me. I put the chickens into crates that held ten birds, struggling to keep the wings down so they wouldn't hurt themselves, yet trying to save myself from their nail-sharp claws.

After I put the chickens into the crates, they immediately quieted down. Finally the pens were empty and our crates were full. In silence we loaded the heavy crates into the pickup truck and headed for the butcher. The sunset shot orange and purple across the building thunderclouds.

We arrived at dusk, the wind whipping up as a thunderstorm crashed overhead, the lightning flashing closer as we transferred the chickens from our crates to the butcher's crates. My arms stung with scratches from their claws. White manure splattered across my sweatshirt and down my overalls. Finally our birds sat quietly in the new crates, ready to sleep now that night had fallen. Tucked under a wide roof overhang, they would be protected from the storm.

The ride home was just as quiet, but I felt an odd mix of pride and relief. We had done it. We had raised a batch of chickens, transported them to the butcher's, and tomorrow Melissa would return to pick them up. Except for the few moments when they'd been crated and re-crated, the chickens lived a calm life on our farm, a life free of chemicals, a life of sunshine and wind and bugs and grass.

At one point on the drive home Melissa reached over and took my hand. "You know, because we've done this tonight, our friends and family will have safe, good-tasting chicken to put in their freezers."

I squeezed her hand. "I know. I just didn't think it would be so hard."

"Me neither," she replied.

The chickens were the warm-up for the truly difficult task of taking lambs to the butcher. I don't want to hurt any poultry-lovers' feelings, but chickens just aren't that attractive, with their beady little eyes and pointed beaks. Mammals, on the other hand, are darned cute.

I learned this the first winter we had lambs on the farm. One blustery morning I was filling the lambs' water trough, my back hunched against the frigid January wind. While we had sold most of the lambs that had been born in the spring to other farmers to raise, enough family and friends had asked to buy lamb to eat that we decided to finish—or raise to market weight—a few lambs. One of those lambs, now seven months old, approached me at the water trough. I waited, incredulous. Unless they've been raised on a bottle, lambs usually want little to do with humans. But this one, his black pupils wide, his ears perked forward, touched my extended mitten.

"Hi, Cutie," I said, lightly tapping his wooly head. But instead of running away, he ducked his head shyly, then looked me in the eye. I tapped him again and he ducked again, moving closer. We played our game for a few minutes while the four other lambs in the pen hung back, nervous. But then my hands froze in midair. What was I doing? This lamb was almost ready for market. In one week this living, breathing, playful lamb would be dead—on purpose. I turned away to shut off the water hydrant. "No, no, no," I muttered. "Leave me alone."

But the lamb, now bold, tugged on my barn coat, tentatively tasting the brown cotton. I watched, horrified, as he presented his head for another tap. He couldn't be a pet. He was already slated to be meat. I suddenly noticed his heart-shaped face, the black spots gently splashed across one ear, his perky tail. How could I pay someone to kill him? I tapped the lamb's head one more time, then fled.

While I knew on an intellectual level that as a farmer I'd be doing this, when you nuzzle baby lamb noses, when you give them shots, when you bury your fingers into wool slick with lanolin, when you *know* the animals, meat takes on a whole new meaning. As the playful lamb's processing date neared, I searched frantically for alternatives, but could find none.

On the scheduled morning we loaded the five sheep into the pickup, a fairly easy task because Mr. Playful followed me up the ramp and the others followed him. We drove the fifteen miles in silence. Melissa backed up to the loading dock and we shooed the sheep into the building's nearest open pen. The holding pens seemed calm enough, but my heart raced nonetheless. A huge cow in the next stall sniffed through the rails. Another sheep, freshly shorn, waited in the pen ahead. I wanted to tap the lamb's head one more time but was too embarrassed to show such affection in front of the man who would kill the lamb. I imagined it would make his job even harder. We closed the heavy wooden door behind us and climbed back into the pickup. Melissa drove around front and went inside to handle the paperwork.

I sat in the pickup and cried. My contacts blurred, my nose filled. Why did I have to face death so directly? Why did everyone else get off free, blissfully ignorant of the death that preceded their meat? I couldn't stop crying. Huge, shuddering sobs. I was still crying when Melissa came out. She held my hand while she drove, and I cried all the way home.

It's easier now, because I've learned so much about being a farmer, and I've given a great deal of thought to why I'm still a carnivore. Before I became a farmer, eating meat was something I did without thought or consideration. It was just food on my plate. Now, however, I'm very conscious that the meat I eat is many things: it's an animal, it's the man or woman who killed and processed the animal, and it's the farmer, or the corporation, who owned and raised the animal.

Also, when I bit into that first bite of lamb from our farm, I was overwhelmed with gratitude . . . gratitude that I'd been able to witness the lamb's life and ensure it was a good one . . . gratitude that the end of its life had come swiftly and without fear . . . gratitude that we had ended up on this piece of land and were feeding people from it.

If raising an animal and taking it to the butcher's is such a hard thing to do, the obvious question is: why raise animals for meat at all? First, I love meat, and the only way most of us are able to eat meat is because a farmer, or a corporation, raised animals. Not to get all noble, but I believe raising food is an important responsibility, one that I can fulfill. I can't fight in the military or be a spiritual leader or an investigative reporter exposing corruption, but I can feed people.

A second reason to raise livestock is that not all land is suited for growing crops. Our land is rolling hills and steep slopes. Drive a tractor long enough on this land, and you and the tractor will end up taking a tumble down the hill. Also, planting most crops disturbs the soil and exposes it to erosion. Wind picks up the soil and swirls it off into the next township. Rain sweeps it down to the bottom of the hill, where it does no one any good. The best way to keep the soil where it belongs is to plant grass. But what's a farmer going to do with hill after hill of grass?

Humans can't digest grass, but grazing animals can, so we put sheep into the pastures and they convert the grass into flesh, which eventually becomes meat.

The third reason might strike people as the oddest, but I continue to farm because I love animals. The irony of this isn't lost on me. You'd think people who raise animals then actually eat them must not like animals very much, but most of the time the exact opposite is true. It's *why* we do what we do. But unless a landowner can afford to keep animals around just to look at (this is called a hobby farm, by the way), the rest of us animal lovers must find a way for the animals to earn their keep and contribute to the economic health of the farm. One of the best ways to do this is to keep sheep or cattle or hogs, get 'em pregnant, then sell the offspring for meat.

As I write this, I am literally surrounded by animals in a grove of box elders that sprang up in the middle of our east pasture. The sheep love this grove, hanging out in the shade or scratching an itch against a tree trunk. Sun filters weakly through the leaves, creating a special haven. One year Melissa suddenly reached up, pulled down a branch, and the ewes came running to munch on the succulent leaves. Now we do it all the time—tree treats.

Not today, though, because I don't want to disturb them, so I sit quietly in my camp chair, ruminating on being a farmer while they ruminate on their cuds of masticated grass. There are about 125 animals within one hundred feet of me, and the only sounds I hear are the traffic from the highway and wind rustling the trees overhead. The ewes are lying down, some lambs stretched out at their sides sound asleep, others chewing their cud. They are content and quiet.

The two-month-old lambs are no longer skinny little things; everything about them is round—round bellies, round thighs, round faces. The farmer in me is proud that we raise such fine animals.

The carnivore in me tries to imagine what will happen in six more months to the lamb standing nearest me, a black-faced guy with long legs and tawny wool. When that lamb is about 120 pounds, a man will stun the lamb into unconsciousness, slit its throat, hang it up by its back legs, peel off its skin, remove its internal organs, cut the carcass up into small pieces, wrap those pieces in clear plastic, label the pieces "chops" and "kabob" and "roast," then I will put the packages in my freezer, eventually thaw one, throw it on the grill with some garlic and rosemary, and I will consume the flesh of the animal before me.

When people find out I farm and raise animals for meat, many smile, shake their heads, and throw their hands up in mock horror. "Just don't remind me that meat's an animal. I don't want to know that."

"Why not?" the farmer in me sputters as I think, *Don't we owe the animals that much?*

The ewes around me stand now, and the lambs also pop to their feet, stretching luxuriantly, then dash over to Mom for a quick milk snack. The families stroll past, eyeing me warily as they head out into the sun to convert more grass into something I can eat: *them.* These animals are content, calm, and happy. A friend calls the meat she buys from us "happy meat." If I'm going to eat animals, these are the ones I want to eat.

When we started farming, we knew it would be very hard to eat an animal we'd named, so we resisted the impulse to name our fifty ewes, but just referred to them by the numbers on their ear tags. All the lambs have only ear tag numbers, not names. Many years later, however, when Melissa calls to ewe "Number 66," that sounds an awful lot like a name. But that's okay, since we don't eat the ewes. We eat their offspring.

People's eyes widen when they learn I eat the lamb meat we raise. I tell them I can eat the animals because the lambs are wild, not pets, and the lambs aren't specifically named individuals.

There are enough of them that when I put my forty pounds of meat in the freezer, it could have been any one of a hundred animals.

Not so with our calf. About the same time we got the wild idea to try raising beef, a four-month-old dairy calf at a friend's farm needed a home. We brought the calf home before we had time to come to our senses. He was a little dark brown cutie, about two hundred pounds, a manageable size if he pushed against you so that you'd scratch his neck. Widen your stance and you could keep your footing.

"Don't name him," I warned Melissa.

"Of course not," she said. We weren't sure if we could actually butcher and eat this guy, but I decided that if we couldn't, we'd keep him around for show. Maybe we'd spray-paint the typical meat cuts on him and use him for educational purposes. We had our bases covered—we wouldn't give him a name, and we had a plan if we couldn't bear to butcher him.

Now, months later, when Melissa approaches the calf's pasture and yells, "Hey, calf!" both I and the calf hear "Calf," not "calf." He comes thundering toward the fence, kicking his heels and tossing his head, totally enamored with Melissa. Tipping the scales at nine hundred pounds, he's a steer now instead of a calf, yet he still wants to push against me for a scratch. I've made the frightening discovery that there is no stance wide enough to withstand the attentions of a nine-hundred-pound steer. Thank god Melissa was there to divert him long enough so that I could flee. Melissa recently confessed that a few times she's even had to scramble over the fence to escape getting hurt. When she brings visitors out to his pasture, he kicks up his heels and whirls in a circle, totally excited. Just our luck to be raising an endearing, dancing steer.

Here's the problem: He's approaching butchering weight. He'll be there in another two months. He has a name. He loves Melissa and she loves him. He cannot stay on the farm, with white dotted lines on his flank showing where steaks and roasts come from, because he's too big, too friendly, and therefore too dangerous. I'm afraid to go into his pen. We can't ask farm-sitters to do this either. He must go for meat.

So when his butcher date arrives, we'll kick ourselves for raising only one steer and becoming attached to him. We'll remember watching him grow and play with the sheep. We'll feel good about the life he's led here—seventeen months of sun and rain and fresh pasture. Then we will load him into the trailer and make that drive.

No matter how much you love your job, I'm sure there are parts of it that are more difficult than others. A livestock farmer's job is to feed people, and part of that job is seeing the process through by killing an animal to make meat. A few weeks after our steer is butchered, ten families will each take home forty pounds of meat, raised with respect and compassion. They won't have met the steer, nor scratched his head, nor watched his happy dances, but that's okay. We've done all that for them, which is why we're farmers in the first place.

# Part Two

# Stuffing Ourselves

We do not eat for the good of living, but because the
meat is savory and the appetite is keen.

—RALPH WALDO EMERSON

M oving sheep can be a tricky business. Basically you encourage them to run away from you in the direction you choose, or you lead them with a bucket of corn. Corn is to sheep what chocolate is to humans.

We needed to run our flock of sixty ewes from the west end of a very long pasture all the way back to the east end. One side of our route was fenced, but the other side was open to more pasture, which might tempt the sheep off the trail. That's when I had a brainstorm. "I'll walk ahead of the sheep with a bucket of corn," I said. "I'll lure them straight ahead, and they'll be so intent on the corn that they won't be tempted to veer off to the left and create chaos. You and the border collie can bring up the rear in case there are stragglers."

I started out about fifty yards ahead of the sheep, and when Melissa opened the fence to let them through, I rattled my bucket of corn as loudly as I could. The lead sheep saw the bucket and heard the rattling, so she headed straight for me and the others followed. This was good.

I began walking, wanting to pace myself since I had about 350 yards to lead the sheep, the length of three and a half football fields. But when I glanced over my shoulder, I noticed the sheep were rapidly closing the distance between us. I broke into an easy jog.

The ground began to shake as the flock approached me at a now alarming rate. The border collie behind them might have had something to do with that.

I began to run. Soon the flock was running right behind me. Then the faster ones ran alongside me. I clutched the bucket to my chest and tried not to think about what would happen if I tripped and fell. Within seconds I was surrounded by sixty frightened sheep that pounded the ground with hard, pointy hooves.

The sheep and I were now all running for our lives, but hey, at least we were running in the right direction. Corn flew from my bucket as my lungs burned and I gasped for air. After running about one hundred yards, I was forced to slow down, sure I'd be run over. Thank god the flock decided my pace wasn't fast enough and moved ahead of me. "Eat our wooly dust," they cried as they thundered past.

Apparently our flock didn't get the memo that sheep are supposed to follow, not lead. Just like my sheep, America likes to think of itself as a leader. We have the highest gross domestic product of any country. We're responsible for the highest percentage of the world's private consumption. We're also in front when it comes to meat consumption. That thundering you hear, however, is the rest of the world stampeding behind us as it follows the rattling bucket full of corn. (If you've read Michael Pollan's *The Omnivore's Dilemma,* you know corn literally drives the modern production of meat.)

On the day I became Woman Who Runs with the Sheep, I learned something important about rattling that bucket of corn and leading the stampede: while a stampede is easy to start, it's very hard to stop, especially if you're in the lead.

# Leading the
# Meat Stampede

... ... ...... ... ...

AS YOU MAY have gathered, I love meat. I grew up eating meat at every meal. For me, meat has always been the main course; everything else is just a side dish. A meal without meat is hollow, like the Tin Man's chest without a heart. The vegetables and bread and salad seem lost and alone, like soldiers who've lost their leader, like the spokes of a wheel that's missing its hub.

Perhaps that's why I've never responded to the pleas of animal rights activists or environmentalists to stop eating meat. I've read book after book about the horrors of factory farming and about how eating meat is cruel and that we should all stop it right now, but I still eat meat, and it's not just because I'm a farmer. I'm not all that interested in the ethics of eating meat, nor the justifications on either side of the debate for whether we should continue eating meat (canine teeth vs. ability to survive without protein from meat, for example). Pro-meat and anti-meat advocates can go at each other all they want about whether eating meat is right or wrong.

One thing is certain: regardless of whether or not we *should* be eating meat, we've been doing it for a very, very long time.

Starting a few million years ago, our predecessors supplemented their grain diets with animals they could catch themselves, or with carcasses stolen from other predators. Then we got smart and began domesticating animals—sheep and goats were the first, ten thousand years ago, then hogs nine thousand years ago, followed by cattle five thousand years ago.

As the world's population grew, meat consumption was tied to wealth—only the privileged ate as much meat as they wanted, and they ate only the better cuts. In medieval Europe most people ate the poorest cuts and boiled the meat to extract every last drop of nutrition. Nobles roasted their meat over direct fire. Since fire was associated with wildness and strength, and strength was connected to power, people who roasted meat believed themselves to be more powerful than those who boiled it.

Today, in developed countries, meat consumption has become much less of a privilege and more of a food that everyone can enjoy. As a result of increased availability and decreasing prices, humans keep consuming more and more meat. Global meat production has increased 500 percent since 1950.[1] According to the International Food Policy Research Institute in Washington, D.C., the fastest increase in consumption is in the developing world, since when people have extra money for food, they buy more meat. Between the 1970s and the 1990s meat consumption in developing countries grew at almost triple the rate consumption grew in industrial countries. The U.N.'s Food and Agriculture Organization estimates the per person annual meat consumption in developing countries rose from twenty-four pounds in 1970 to sixty-four pounds in 2002.[2]

That brings today's meat consumption in the developing world up to about *half* of what Americans were eating . . . nearly sixty years ago. In the 1950s the average American meat consumption was 138 pounds per year. In the 1970s this rose to 177 pounds.

Of this 177 pounds, 42 percent was beef, 36 percent pork, 16 percent chicken, and 7 percent was veal and lamb.[3]

By 2005 our consumption had increased to 200 pounds per person. (Other sources claim we hit 220 pounds by 2005, but I'll stick with the USDA numbers to be consistent, since *everyone's* a magician when it comes to statistics.) Beef took a hit, falling to 36 percent, pork fell to 27 percent, veal and lamb dropped to below 1 percent (a hard figure for this shepherd to stomach), but chicken shot into first place, now 37 percent of the meat we eat.[4]

We eat much more meat than the citizens of other developed countries. As the Worldwatch Institute so succinctly put it in a headline: "United States Leads World Meat Stampede." According to the institute, Germans eat 189 pounds of meat per person per year; Italians, 180 pounds; Argentinians, 176 pounds; and Americans lead the pack with 270 pounds.[5] This figure is 70 pounds higher than the USDA figure, so it raises a few questions. Are we underestimating? Are they overestimating? Or are we somewhere in between? Whichever estimate is more accurate, the fact remains that Americans are consuming a great deal of meat.

Both consumption and production amounts in developing countries are fast on our heels. The International Food Policy Research Institute expects a 50 percent increase in China's meat consumption by 2020 and a 40 percent increase in Southeast Asia. Africa's demand is expected to double.[6]

Americans will continue to lead this stampede. The USDA projects our annual meat consumption will be 220 pounds by 2016.[7] From my standpoint as a farmer, that's wonderful. In fact, perhaps some of that 220 pounds could even end up including a few pounds of the lamb I raise. (We shepherds are mighty optimists.)

We're heading for 220 pounds per person every year, but what does that really mean? Pounds per year seems sort of distant from my life as a farmer and is difficult for me to visualize. That's why I found so interesting the calculation Michael W. Fox included in his 1997 book, *Eating with Conscience.* He converted the number of animals killed every year into a person's lifetime consumption of animals. According to Fox, in 1997 the meat industry was butchering 7,000 calves, 130,000 cattle, 360,000 hogs, and 24 million chickens every day. Wow. He then came up with an estimate of how many animals an American would eat in his or her lifetime. His result was 2,400 animals, which would be about 30 animals a year if we live to the age of eighty.[8]

I know Fox wants me to be shocked by this number, but I find it interesting. I don't know why his number is more helpful than 220 pounds per year, but it is. It's concrete. It shifts the focus from meat as a per pound product to meat as an animal.

Since so much time has passed since these figures were calculated, I decided to update them. Because Fox didn't explain how he reached his 2,400 figure, I was unable to duplicate his methods exactly, so I went about it my own way and arrived at the crude estimate of 2,500 animals killed per person in a lifetime.[9]

This number is obviously skewed, since it assumes we eat the same amount of meat at every age, but I'm guessing a three-year-old won't be downing the same number of steaks and burgers that a forty-year-old will. Also, this number *grossly* overstates consumption, since humans do not consume all of a slaughtered animal. These problems don't bother me, however, because complete accuracy isn't the point here.

The point is that at age fifty I'm five-eighths of the way through my expected life, which means about 1,560 animals have already been raised and killed on my behalf. There's nothing I can do about the choices I've made regarding those animals. It's the remaining 940 that concern me.

# How Much
# Is Too Much?

••• ••• •••••• ••• •••

WHETHER WE LOOK at our annual meat consumption as 220 pounds or as 30 animals, it's hard to avoid the next two questions: why are we eating more meat, and are we eating too much?

Experts tend to agree that we're consuming more because meat is cheaper than ever before. We're also cooking less, instead relying on convenience food and restaurants to feed us. According to the U.S. Food and Drug Administration (FDA), Americans now spend nearly half of their food budgets on food "prepared away from home," and we get 32 percent of our calories from this food.[10]

Eating out means larger portions because everything has been supersized. The *American Journal of Public Health* lists the evidence: "Restaurants are using larger dinner plates, bakers are selling larger muffin tins, pizzerias are using larger pans, and fast-food companies are using larger drink and French fry containers."[11] Automobile manufacturers are installing larger cup holders in cars. Cookie recipes in new editions of *Joy of Cooking* yield fewer cookies than identical recipes in the old editions because we make our cookies larger now. We used to drop a teaspoon of dough onto the cookie sheet, but now we drop big, generous tablespoons that bake down into monster cookies.

According to the USDA, our portions are much larger than necessary. In a Clemson University survey of restaurants, 27 percent of the chefs served four ounces of pasta, 32 percent served six-ounce servings, and 18 percent filled the plate with eight ounces.[12] The spoilsports at the USDA say two ounces is plenty.

The USDA recommends four ounces of meat, yet 28 percent of chefs served eight-ounce steaks, and nearly 50 percent weighed down their plates with twelve-ounce steaks. A steak today is 224 percent larger than the USDA believes it needs to be.

Upscale restaurants are starting to reduce portion size and use smaller plates. I visited a trendy San Francisco restaurant filled with professional types dressed in black, moss green, and khaki suits, and bravely ordered something exotic—what, I can't remember.

What I do remember is the sinking feeling when the plate arrived—a small, gleaming white plate with even smaller food portions. Great. I'd be paying three times as much money for about one-third the amount of food I was used to on my plate. It was amazing how quickly that value response kicked in. Yet by the end of the meal, I wasn't faint from hunger or too weak to walk back to my hotel, but very satisfied.

Eating meat is more than just a way to meet your protein requirements. Meat has even become a way to communicate your personality while on a date. The *New York Times* reported that women have begun embracing ordering meat when on a date, now believing that ordering salads displays an "unappealing mousiness." Choosing a steak, on the other hand, sends the message to your date that you're "unpretentious and down to earth and unneurotic." As the *Times* said, "I am woman, hear me chew."[13]

As our consumption increases in size, so do we. More than 64 percent of us are considered overweight, and more than 30 percent are obese, according to the FDA. Medical expenditures linked to weight issues now reach $92.6 billion per year, more than 9 percent of total U.S. medical expenditures.

There's no denying we love food, and meat, and lots of it. In 2004 a Salt Lake City couple on the Atkins diet—no carbs, but loads of meat—was banned from Chuck-A-Rama's all-you-can-eat buffet because they were eating nothing on the buffet but the meat, and lots of it. After the man returned to the carving board for his *twelfth* slice of roast beef, the chef asked him to stop.[14] Cripes, why did he wait that long? Seems that even six slices of roast beef qualifies as excessive, but that's just me.

Trying to find out how much meat we actually *need* is to step into the fray between animal rights activists, vegetarian organizations, nutritionists, and meat promotional groups, since they all promote their own agendas with scientific research proving we need, or don't need, animal protein. Since this is the sort of debate that once again makes my ganglia twitch, I decided to sidestep it and go straight to the USDA to find out what they think I should be putting into my mouth.

Yes, I realize Uncle Sam might have a bias as well, but I just wanted a basic guideline to determine where today's annual two hundred pounds of meat consumption falls in the continuum between "No Meat" and "Way Too Much Meat." I Googled the term "food pyramid" and found the USDA's Web site: http:// mypyramid.gov. I entered my height, weight, gender, age, and level of physical exercise so the site could tell me how much meat I should be eating.

The USDA apparently can't resist commenting on your weight. Before the Web site gave me my suggested daily consumption levels, the site flashed up this screen: "Please note: The weight you entered is above the healthy range for your height.

Would you like to choose a food plan for your current weight [and die a horrible, premature death as a total lard bucket—or at least that's what I read between the lines], or choose a plan to gradually move toward a healthier weight?"

*Butt out,* I thought, so I chose "plan for current weight." Here's what I should be eating every day: 8 ounces of grains, 3 cups of vegetables, 2 cups of fruit, 3 cups of milk, and 6.5 ounces of meat and beans. Just for ducks, I checked the plan for gradually moving toward a "healthier weight," and the daily meat suggestion was 5.5 ounces.

Eating 6.5 ounces of meat every day adds up to about 148 pounds a year. At 200 pounds per year, I'm eating 35 percent more than the U.S. government thinks I should be eating. I found a few vegetarian Web sites that claimed we're eating 300–500 percent more protein than we need. (See why this is so confusing?) If I want to take the pyramid's recommendation to slim down, I should be eating only about 125 pounds of meat per year.

Studies abound showing that too much animal fat is hard on our hearts and arteries, which is probably what's behind MyPyramid's suggestion to eat only lean or low-fat meat, and to not eat that much. Yet most of us tend to ignore the dietary guidelines and the warnings. One enthusiastic food blogger explained why: "We're Americans! Of course we eat poorly! We're the home of McDonald's, Chef-boy-Ardee, and ConAgra. Bad eating is in our blood."

The *Smithsonian* gathered together some amazing statistics to show that Americans are "livin' large." The average U.S. adult weighed 10 percent more in 2003 than in the 1980s. In 1976 only three NFL players weighed more than 300 pounds; in 2006 more than 500 players tipped the scales at 300. The standard movie seat expanded from 19 to 22 inches, and the standard casket has been bumped out 4 inches to today's 26 inches. In 1950 the average house provided 290 square feet per inhabitant. Now we've got almost 900 square feet of elbow room for each family member in the house.[15]

This list does give one pause. When we reach our projected per person consumption of 220 pounds of meat in 2016, only eight years from now, will the movie seats and caskets be forced to bump out again? Do we really need to eat this much meat? At what point do we decide we're eating too much?

# Listen to Your Mother
# and Clean Up Your Plate

••• ••• •••••• ••• •••

ANOTHER THING TO consider when you sit down to eat is how much of that meat you will throw away. The USDA Economic Research Service (ERS) put out a report in 1997 that attempted to quantify the amount of food that is wasted or thrown away in this country. It focused on what it called "plate loss," or the food that never makes it from our plates into our mouths. Plate loss happens in the food-service industry—restaurants—and at home.

The common sources of food-service plate loss are: overpreparation of menu items; expanded menu choices, which can make it harder to manage food inventories; unexpected fluctuations in food sales due to sudden changes in the weather or other factors; and the upsizing of food portions. And unless consumers take home the uneaten food on their plate, it must be thrown away.

Plate loss at home is similar—we didn't plan right, and something spoiled in the refrigerator. Or we didn't eat everything on our plate and threw the rest away.

Of the 96 billion pounds of edible food that was "lost" in 1995, meat, poultry, and fish accounted for 8.2 billion pounds. Divide this by 365 and it means we're throwing away 22.5 million pounds of meat every day. Those figures are from ten years ago.[16]

Once I've created a product—meat—and sold it to a customer, what that customer does with it is out of my hands. I've been paid, and as long as the customer is satisfied with the service and quality of my product, I don't have any expectations other than to hope the customer returns. If that customer wants to eat one bite of a lamb chop and throw the rest away (which he won't, because our lamb tastes great), that's his business. So as a farmer, I can do nothing about plate loss. But it does irk me, and I'm not the only one.

All-you-can-eat buffets must bring the worst out in us. Employees of a Chinese buffet in Des Moines, Iowa, had been watching a woman and her family on previous trips to the restaurant and were fed up with her habits, disgusted that these people would take one bite out of an egg roll then throw it away, or take four pieces of crab rangoon and eat only one. So the next time the woman visited and did the same thing again, management snapped and asked her to leave. The Dragon House manager said his restaurant offers an all-you-can-*eat* buffet, not all-you-can-*waste*.[17] The woman was embarrassed to have been scolded, but perhaps this is what some people need—to have someone else notice how much they are wasting and call them on it.

In one two-week period I witnessed two horrendous examples of waste. I attended a one-hundred-dollar-per-plate fund-raiser for a local literary organization, and the caterer must have felt that people needed a great deal of food on their plates for that price. Waiters delivered plates of food to more than five hundred people. Alongside the prerequisite soggy vegetables, each plate contained four thick slices of beef and a very large herb-stuffed chicken breast. I stared down at my plate. This was a ridiculous amount of meat, and I doubted anyone could eat all of it.

I was right. At the end of the dinner, I scanned the plates around me and saw that everyone had either eaten all of the chicken and none of the beef, half of each, or all of the beef and none of the chicken. A friend sitting at a nearby table was so horrified to think that so much meat was to be thrown away that she "borrowed" a plate and filled it full of meat to take home to her dogs.

At a writing conference I attended the following week, meals were included in the price, which meant there was no way to opt out if you had other plans. As a result, the caterers prepared meals for more people than ever intended to eat them, and they were pleading with people to return to the buffet table for seconds and thirds. I shudder at what must have been thrown away, not because of the cost, but because animals were killed for nothing. And this was just in my little corner of the world.

I contribute my own share to the 22.5 million pounds of food waste. Just last week, in a totally stupid, brain-fart, junior-moment sort of screw-up, I made a chicken-and-pea-pod stir-fry using as my thickener, not the correct cornstarch, but baking soda. (Please don't laugh—it's humiliating enough just to admit this.) Baking soda doesn't thicken; instead it turns the peas black and makes the chicken taste like ammonia (as reported by the brave Melissa). We had to throw the entire pot out. I wasted two fist-fuls of pea pods and two very large chicken breasts.

The pea pods had come from the neighbor's garden, and I'm sorry to have wasted them, but the lost pea pods didn't upset me as much as the one pound of lost chicken. I'd purchased the boneless, skinless breasts from Lori and Al, our friends (and Melissa's employer). They had purchased the chicken as a one-day-old chick and put it in a brooding building to keep it warm with a few hundred other baby chicks. When the chicken was a few weeks old, it was moved into a larger building with screens for walls, so there was plenty of air circulation and some sun but no danger from predators. The chicken had eaten heartily for another four weeks, then been moved into a small crate and driven fifty feet to the back of the processing building.

Once inside the building, an employee named Andrew picked up the bird and put it upside down in a cone, which immobilized it so it couldn't flap around in fright. Then he cut its throat and waited for the chicken's blood to drain entirely from the body so that the blood wouldn't discolor the meat. The dead chicken was dunked in scalding hot water to loosen the feathers, then put in an automatic plucker. Someone cut off the head and legs and then passed the carcass down to Melissa, who cut open the carcass and pulled out the internal organs. A State of Minnesota meat inspector stood nearby, inspecting each and every carcass and its organs. The carcass was cut up into pieces. The breast meat was deboned and deskinned. Eugene put the meat on a tray, and Loraine covered it with plastic wrap and used the heat machine to seal the wrap. Molly weighed the package and slapped a label on it. I paid money for the two breasts, so Lori and Al were compensated for all that went into raising and processing those two chicken breasts. That's how capitalism works.

But still, I couldn't shake my horror that a chicken had died just so I could waste a good share of that chicken. That's when I decided to once again take up Michael Fox's approach to converting pounds of meat consumed to animals eaten, only this time I would convert pounds of meat wasted every day, 22.5 million pounds, into animals.

I ran the numbers, and here's what I came up with: every day we are killing then completely throwing away 15,000 cattle, 36,000 hogs, and 2 million chickens.[18]

That's every day.

No one, *no one,* can feel good about these numbers.

Let's say my calculations are crude and unsophisticated, since they are. A real economist would use econometrics and calculus and statistical data for the last fifteen years to build an equation as long as my arm, and *then* run the numbers. Since I'm no longer a real economist, let's cut my estimate in half to be on the safe side. Now we are throwing away only 7,500 cattle, 18,000 hogs, and 1 million chickens a day.

Somehow I don't feel any better. Throwing away 7,500 cows every day just isn't something that I, as a carnivore, can get behind.

What will it take for us to start paying more attention to the fact that the food we are buying and throwing away is an animal? The folks at Meatpaper, a new online journal that focuses on all things meat, interviewed San Francisco chef Chris Cosentino and asked him if he felt compassion toward the animals he served. Here's his answer:

> About two years ago I took my entire kitchen crew, three cooks, and food writer Harold McGee, and we went down and did a goat slaughter, which would later go into an Easter supper at my house. We bought the goats and slaughtered them on the farm. And I'll tell you, from that day on, there were never any mistakes with meat in this restaurant. . . . [T]he cooks that watched the slaughter . . . realized that there's an animal dying. There needs to be that consciousness in this industry. . . . And it was hard. It was really hard. I don't think people realize what it does to you emotionally. It makes you really think about what you're doing at the restaurant every day.[19]

Carnivores who pay attention can increase their Compassion Quotient by simply wasting less meat. This is the easiest step a meat eater can take.

Jonathan Bloom's blog (http://wastedfood.com) gives ideas on how to stop throwing away so much food, and shares what other people have tried. For example, at one college a few brave souls took up posts at the cafeteria trash cans and began eating off the other students' plates to show how much food they were leaving on those plates. A Maine college did away with its cafeteria trays, and food waste dropped from five ounces per student to three. Students aren't wasting as much food because they can't carry as much without the trays—and they end up satisfied with what they've eaten, so they don't return for more.

All of this is common sense, but when you look at our food waste, clearly this sort of sense isn't as common as it once was. When you cook at home, make sure you use leftovers before they go bad. Cook smaller portions if you don't like leftovers. Use smaller plates. When you're at a restaurant, order only what you know you can eat. Take the leftovers home and eat them; don't let them turn into a mold experiment in the back of your fridge. Split an order of prime rib or chicken Alfredo instead of each ordering your own meal and letting half go to waste. Ask your server for half portions. I've started ordering from the appetizer menu and find the portions are just fine. I'm full, I clean up my plate, and I'm not throwing any animals into the trash can.

When I was a kid, Mom told me to clean up my plate because there were starving children in Africa who didn't have what I had. Do parents still do this today? Did it become children in Darfur or Bosnia? As an adult, although I know that cleaning up my plate won't directly help starving children in Africa, I do know it's still the right thing to do. If we're going to kill millions of animals every year for food, the least we can do is respect those animals by actually eating them. Throwing meat away is, well, a waste.

We'll all do better to take smaller portions, plan our meals more carefully, clean up our plates just like Mom nagged us to, and never thicken our stir-fry sauce with baking soda.

## Part Three

# Old MacDonald's Farm
# Is Gone, e–i–e–i–o

"Get big or get out."

—ADVICE TO FARMERS FROM EZRA TAFT BENSON,
U.S. SECRETARY OF AGRICULTURE FROM 1953 TO 1961

While wasting less meat is a step I can easily take, I do tend to get my hackles up whenever animal rights activists and the more vocal vegetarians try to convince me I must give up meat altogether in order to be an ethical, moral, and kind person. I've come across nearly a dozen books in which authors first rail about the effects of modern agriculture on the environment and how irresponsible we are to let it continue, then come to the conclusion we must therefore all stop eating meat. Even though I agree with many of their points, it really gets my knickers in a twist when someone tries to tell me what to eat.

Maybe if a *carnivore* had delivered the same message to me years ago, I might have listened, but I didn't. So when I started really paying attention to how our modern meat-production system works, it was a bit of a kick in the teeth to discover that those darned animal rights activists and vocal vegetarians just might be on to something— factory farming is bad, bad, bad. It's the *solution* as to what's to be done about it—that's where some of us might differ.

My look into farming and our food system revealed a discomforting fact: Old MacDonald's farm was no longer feeding me, so it was time to pay closer attention to who—or what—*was* feeding me.

An old-fashioned technique for getting rid of all sorts of nasty parasites on a sheep or cow, such as scab mites, blowflies, ticks, keds, and lice, was to fill a tank with a liquid formula of water, insecticide, and fungicide. The liquid, at least for sheep, was called sheep dip. (An interesting side note that may or may not be related: in the days of bootleg whiskey, moonshiners would call their product "sheep dip" to avoid paying liquor taxes, and today there's a Scotch whiskey called Sheep Dip.)

The sheep or cow would be herded down into a long, narrow tub filled with sheep dip (or cattle dip), deep enough that the animal would have to swim. Then a guy with a pole would walk along the tub and briefly push the animal's head all the way under the water, thereby making sure insects on the animal's body couldn't use the head as an island. The animal then reached underwater steps leading up and out of the tub, and emerged free of pests. I would imagine that this experience, although brief, must have been harrowing and not much fun for the animal.

Our look at modern agriculture will be much the same: brief, a bit harrowing, and not much fun. Sorry about that.

# Falling for
# Little Bo Peep

... ... ...... ... ...

MOST OF US urban types grew up with an image of the farm created by children's books with the ubiquitous red barn, two hogs,
two sheep, two cows, and a farmer wearing overalls and a straw
hat. We, or our children, spent hours with a Fisher-Price plastic red
barn, red silo, and little plastic animals, and the little plastic
farmer, once again in overalls and hat. We learned animal sounds
by singing about Old MacDonald's farm, on which you'd find a
diverse range of animals—an oink-oink here, a moo-moo there.

We recited the nursery rhyme about Little Bo Peep, who'd
somehow lost her sheep. Our mothers sang to us about Little Boy
Blue, the boy whose animals were out of control—the sheep in
the meadow, the cows in the corn—because he was fast asleep
under the haystack. These rhymes not only shaped our childhood
images of farms, but they also prove that young children shouldn't
be put in charge of livestock. Today I know that if those cows
spend too much time marauding through the cornfield, they'll
probably bloat up and die.

We believe that good, wholesome people live on farms and lead good, wholesome lifestyles that produce good, wholesome food. Our wistful connection to farms, a life *not* lived by 99.3 percent of this country's population, comes through even in our responses to homes. The very image of a farmhouse packs a great deal of emotional impact into its white siding and welcoming front porch. Environmental psychologist Jack Nasar studied the symbolic language of homes by showing people sketches of six types of homes and asking them which they'd approach for help if they had a flat tire. Of the six styles—Mediterranean, Colonial, Tudor, contemporary, Cape Cod, and farmhouse—the participants overwhelmingly preferred the farmhouse, because it said "friendly."[1]

Agribusiness marketing professionals want us to retain this iconic but out-of-touch-with-reality image of a farm, and they do their best to keep us in the past by putting green grass and red barns on food labels, thereby triggering the same sense of trust and comfort that makes people choose a farmhouse over a Colonial-style house. Writer Kim Severson calls it greenwashing, a genre of food packaging designed to make sure manufacturers "grab their slice of the $25 billion that American shoppers spend each year on natural or organic food." Severson lists the essential elements: "Start with a gentle image of a field or a farm to suggest an ample harvest gathered by an honest, hard-working family. To that end, strangely oversize vegetables or fruits are good. . . . A little red tractor is O.K. Pesticide tanks and rows of immigrant farm laborers bent over in the hot sun are not."[2]

Unfortunately, because we stopped paying attention, we've been duped into believing the small, gentle farms of our youth still exist, and we are unwilling to give up our quaint image of Old MacDonald's farm, with chickens pecking in the barnyard and a rooster crowing at dawn (they crow all day, by the way).

Drive through most rural areas in this country, especially the Midwest, and you'll see lots of iconic big red barns. At the sight of these barns, most reasonable people might safely assume that small farms are alive and well.

Look closer. Is there a fence around the barn? No fence *around* the barn means no animals *in* the barn. People moved off the farm in droves during the twentieth century, so most of those nice red barns are not actually being used to raise animals. As we'll see, the animals moved off the farm as well.

Learning about farms takes a meat eater right to the source, giving you the knowledge you need to wade through those choices we all face—factory or small farm, feedlot or pasture, organic or not, local or not. A carnivore's most important tool for making better choices is a clear-eyed view of today's farms—what they are, and what they can be. To get that clear-eyed view, we need to take a peek back about sixty years.

For decades farms didn't change much. As yet untouched by technology, farmers raised a variety of both crops and livestock, providing food for their families and selling the rest. I found a charming 1920 book on farming called *Farm Animals*. The book's language sounds quaint today, but the message comes through loud and clear. The authors, Thomas Forsyth Hunt and Charles William Burkett, took a stab at explaining the role farm animals played in people's lives in 1920: "Whether kept merely as pets and companions, or for the production of work, clothing and food, [animals] compel habits of care and responsibility and inculcate habits of mercy. These habits, together with the sympathetic influences involved, in all ages have had and still continue to have, an elevating and civilizing influence upon the human race."[3]

Habits of care. Habits of responsibility. Habits of mercy. I love these phrases. They are phrases we can all practice, not just farmers.

After World War II, however, Hunt and Burkett's farm began changing when agriculture was swept up in the country's modernization fever. The old ways were outdated; the new ways were modern and the only way to go. During the 1930s and 1940s, when my grandparents ran a flock of six hundred ewes on their southeastern Montana ranch, everything happened outside. The six hundred sheep gave birth to their lambs out on the range. Only the hardiest, the best, and most efficient sheep survived to pass that toughness on to their lambs. My grandmother left the ranch in the 1950s, letting a brother run it, and by the time she'd returned in the early 1960s, modern agriculture had arrived, and only hopelessly out-of-touch, old-fashioned shepherds continued with the old-fashioned model. Suddenly sheep needed to be brought into the barn, fussed over, treated like animals too stupid to know how to care for their own babies. Don't get me started.

A Wisconsin farmer, Ginger Quick, recalls her childhood on the farm: "I remember when the agricultural agents and chemical companies started pushing the farms around here to get bigger. They kept saying, 'You've got to have a bulk tank. You've got to make your barn bigger. You've got to milk more cows. You've got to rent more land.' My dad didn't have a lot of faith in agricultural agents and chemical companies. He said, 'No, I'm not going into debt.' And he kept small."[4]

"Get bigger or get out" became the mantra of modern farming, and Ginger's dad ended up in the minority because most farmers elected to get big. They brought animals in off pasture, put them in feedlots, and kept them there. Bought larger and more powerful tractors. Farmed huge tracts of land. Narrowed their focus, raising fewer types of crops, fewer types of livestock. Then, thanks to the crushing debt loads associated with getting bigger, many farmers who got big also ended up getting out in the mid-1980s because they lost their farms to creditors. For many farmers, agriculture secretary Ezra Taft Benson's urge to "get big or get out" turned into "get big *and* get out."

In 1900, 60 percent of the U.S. population lived on farms and produced food.[5] Farmers were 38 percent of the labor force.[6] There were 5.7 million farms, with an average size of 147 acres. By 1990 farmers comprised 2.6 percent of the labor force. The number of farms dropped to 2.1 million, with an average size of 461 acres.

By 1990 less than 2 percent of the population farmed. Today that figure is .7 percent, less than 1 percent of the population.[7] I thought being a lesbian put me in a tiny minority, but that's nothing compared to the minuscule number of farmers. It's impossible to know exactly how many Americans are gay or lesbian, but the figures currently tossed around are that 3 percent of the country's population are gay women, and 7 percent are gay men. This means there are more than four times as many lesbians as farmers, and ten times as many gay men as farmers. I don't include this useless factoid to upset anyone, since it's not like we'll be taking over the world anytime soon, but I find it a bit unnerving to think that so few people are feeding so many.

To discuss sizes of farms involves a frightening descent into the world of the USDA Economic Research Service, which puts out more charts and tables every year than I, for one, care to read. To sift through them for bits of information gives me a bad case of Information Overload.

Carnivores don't need all that. What we do need is a basic understanding that the best measurement of farm size isn't acreage, it's sales and income. Small farms are those with annual sales below $250,000, and because more than 70 percent of the farms larger than five hundred acres make less than $250,000, they are classified as small farms.[8] Farms with sales less than $10,000 now account for half of all U.S. farms. This is why on most farms there will be no one home during the day to help you with that flat tire. Many farmers need off-farm jobs to survive.

The big guys, the ones the USDA calls "large family farms," "very large family farms," and "nonfamily farms," make up 8 percent of the total but account for 68 percent of total farm production. These farms are cranking out a lot of product. But watch out for the phrase "family farm," which implies small and cozy. The USDA says that 98 percent of this country's farms are family farms—sole proprietorships, partnerships, or family corporations.[9] "Family" does not mean "small."

I think of farms not only in terms of sales, but also in terms of how they operate. Most U.S. farms are conventional farms. It's a bit difficult to describe the modern, conventional farm, because it can range from small to huge, from no livestock to lots of livestock, from a diverse cropping system to the monoculture of raising only one or two crops. Animals are finished using some combination of grain and hay, possibly pasture. The conventional farmer applies pesticides and herbicides to his crops and spreads chemical nitrogen onto his fields as fertilizer. The animals might be given growth hormones and antibiotics so that they'll grow faster and stay healthier in the feedlot. There may be employees, or the farmer may do all the work. The farmer owns or rents the land and the buildings, owns the animals, and chooses what to feed those animals and how to raise them.

Most conventional farms have feedlots. They usually sell their animals at the livestock market or directly to meat companies as a commodity, an agricultural product sold without distinguishing between individual producers. For example, all the corn in an area is brought to the grain elevator, loaded together, and sold simply as corn. A livestock farmer will sell his hogs under contract to a pork company, and those hogs become part of the company's supply of pork. A cattle rancher will sell his cattle at a livestock market, where they're purchased to become part of the country's beef supply. Most farm products are sold as commodities; a farmer's alternative is to market her products directly to consumers, thereby staying completely out of the commodity stream, selling a product specifically identified with her farm. For example, when we sell our lambs to another farmer to finish, that lamb will become part of the commodity stream of lamb. If we sell our lamb directly to Deb or Emily or Jan, it's Rising Moon Farm lamb, a product tied specifically to our farm. Most conventional farmers probably don't sell many animals directly to consumers and aren't set up to do that.

In my township I'm surrounded by conventional farmers, and they're swell people. My North Dakota uncle and aunt are conventional, a Montana aunt and uncle are conventional, and a late Montana uncle was conventional. This may seem obvious, but it's important to separate any judgment about farms from a judgment about farmers. Conventional farmers have fed us for decades. They are businesspeople trying to support themselves and their families just like the rest of us. Because they are engaged in food production is no reason farmers should nobly sacrifice a decent living or their children's college education to do so. Farmers are no more responsible for the state of agriculture today than a nurse is responsible for the complicated health care system, or an autoworker is responsible for the decline in Detroit's share of the automobile market. Over the years farmers made individual choices for their specific farms based on what university researchers were telling them, based on what seed and chemical agribusiness companies were selling them, and—here's where we come in—based on what you and I, the consumers, were willing to pay for meat.

Those conventional farms kept growing larger and larger until some corporation went wild and began using the Widget Theory of Production. When I was in college, professors and textbooks demonstrated economic theory by using the example of a widget factory. A widget was a made-up product, but today there actually are widgets, and they have something to do with computers, but I'm sticking with the nonreal widget, which is some sort of undefined thing.

Let's say I'm an entrepreneur with a widget-making factory. To make my widgets I bring together land (where the building sits), labor (my employees), and inputs (all the little pieces I need to build my widget). If I'm clever about combining those three things, I'll produce lots of widgets as cheaply as possible, people will buy them, and I'll make a profit. Isn't economics grand?

If I can make more widgets using the same amount of land, I've achieved some cost savings, or economies of scale, by lowering my land cost per widget. If I can speed up my workers so that they produce more widgets in the same amount of time, that means more economies of scale, because I've lowered my labor cost per widget. Anytime I can increase my profit without increasing my expenses by the same amount, I'll realize some economies of scale.

Modern agriculture has achieved astronomical economies of scale when it comes to raising meat. Instead of housing a handful of laying hens in a small barn and letting them roam the barnyard during the day, you construct a building over that barnyard, stack the hens in cages inside, and suddenly your egg production goes through the roof. You realize a much higher profit than if you'd just let those original hens do their thing.

Keep growing larger, and when you pass the magic number (usually a thousand head of cattle, twenty-five hundred hogs, or a hundred thousand chickens), then, *voilà*, you've got yourself a factory farm.[10] The actual term for this supersized "farm" is CAFO: concentrated animal feeding operation. Confined Animal Feeding Operation also works, as does Cruel Animal Feeding Operation. Callous Animal Feeding Operation. Someone stop me.

Want to produce more widgets? Cram more widget parts into the factory and speed up the production line. Want more meat?

Cram more animals into the CAFO and put weight on them faster and more cheaply.

One problem, and it's a big one: a cow is not a widget. Neither is a pig or a beef steer or a chicken. They need to eat, drink, and defecate, and their quality of life will certainly deteriorate if there are fifty thousand animals in the pen with them instead of fifty, or if they are kept in cages or feedlots instead of allowed to move around. Yet modern agriculture sees them as nothing more than factory parts used to put together widgets called chicken Alfredo or beef Wellington or pork roast. There is a cost associated with treating animals this way, but that cost isn't borne by the company, it's borne by the animals themselves. When a business creates a cost but makes someone—or something—else pay for it, this is called an externality. The cost is external, or outside, of the business itself.

For example, let's say the process I use to produce widgets creates lots of wastewater, and I don't want to spend the money to remove pollutants from the water. I release it untreated, and the pollutants make their way into your streams and rivers and groundwater. Now you must pay someone to filter your water before you drink it. Oops. Sorry about that. But since the water is on your property, not mine, I don't have to pay your filtering costs. It's external to my business.

Or let's say my widget-making factory really creates a stink, and this horrible smell drifts through the air a few miles and into your house. You feel sick a lot, but that's not my fault. You try to sell the house, but because my factory makes living in your house so unpleasant, the value of the house falls by forty thousand dollars, and you lose that money. Once again, my bad, but it's your house, your problem, and external to my business.

This is fun, so let's keep going. What if my widgets are edible? I want to make them as cheaply as possible, so I pump them full of chemicals, some of which might be carcinogenic. You eat lots and lots of my widgets, develop cancer, are sick and out of work for two years, and must spend one hundred thousand dollars of your own money on medical costs. Not to keep repeating myself, but . . . not my problem. I didn't force you to eat my widgets. And if you eat so many widgets that you gain weight and have a heart attack, or your knee breaks down and you need a new one, tsk, tsk. Not my fault you have no willpower. I am not responsible. That's because I'm a corporation, and as everyone knows, we're not about responsibility, we're about profit.

Thanks to the ability of factory farms to push some of the costs of production off onto the animals, the environment, and people, we've been paying prices for meat that are below the actual costs of producing it. You're not paying for the externalities . . . someone else is.

So while we've been asleep at the wheel, secure in the cozy belief that our meat is being raised by Little Bo Peep and Little Boy Blue on Old MacDonald's farm, something else entirely different has grown up in its place. This something different is a place few humans see unless they work there, but it's where billions of animals spend every hour of every day for most of their short lives.

# It's *Not*
# a Wonderful Life

... ... ...... ... ...

AFTER OBSERVING MY animals for many years, here's what I think comprises a quality life for a livestock animal: the right kind of food, and plenty of it; fresh water; lots of room to run and exercise; fresh air free from stink and airborne diseases; and the freedom to engage in instinctive behaviors. Pets, wild animals, and livestock animals all have these needs.

What happens when those needs aren't met? Hunt and Burkett, my 1920 farm authors, nailed it: "Where the sun does not enter, the physician does."[11] Animals pay a pretty hefty share of the modern system's externalities through their quality of life.

Anyone with a cat or dog (or horse or guinea pig or ferret or African parrot) knows that animals have emotions and definite likes and dislikes and needs. Livestock are no different in their emotional needs. However, there's an additional factor when it comes to considering the life of meat animals. What they eat, how they live, what drugs they're given, their stresses, and how they're killed are all factors that affect their bodies, their muscles.

We *eat* those muscles, our stomachs break them down, and our bodies absorb those animals. It's taken me years, and a farm, to finally link a livestock animal's life with my own.

The best way to approach factory farming is to take a brief look at the lives of each type of animal, from the chicken to the pig to the cow. While eggs and dairy products aren't meat, they come from animals whose lives are just as affected by our food purchases as meat animals. Also, chickens and dairy animals end up in the meat supply eventually.

Let's start small, with hens bred for laying eggs (these hens are called layers). Of the eggs we buy in the store or at a restaurant, 98 percent come from chickens crammed up to nine in a cage, one hundred thousand hens to a building.[12] They never see the sun, never chase grasshoppers, never take dust baths in loose soil, and they have their beaks trimmed so that they don't peck each other to death out of boredom. Hens kept inside do not remain healthy, so they are kept alive with antibiotics until they've produced enough eggs to be considered profitable. When their production falls, they are denied food for up to two weeks to force them to molt, the process whereby they drop their feathers, grow more, and then start laying eggs again. (A hen molts naturally once a year.) After a year or two of this, the chicken is worn out and is sold for meat.

Factory farms know that cramming chickens into a cage stresses them out, so they have turned to science for help, which hasn't let them down in the past. As author Roger Horowitz has pointed out, although scientists can do little to change the gestation periods from fertilization to birth, "virtually every other aspect of animal growth and reproduction fell under the lens of science and technological experimentation."[13] Scientists are currently working to alter the DNA of caged animals, looking for the gene that causes stress so that they can remove it.[14] Perhaps the large poultry companies think if they can genetically alter a hen so that it doesn't *mind* being crammed tightly into a cage, then we consumers can relax and stop worrying about factory farming.

I wrote a children's picture book called *The Perfect Nest,* about a cat named Jack who built the perfect nest to attract the perfect chicken, who would lay a perfect egg for Jack to eat. As is typical in picture books, Jack's plan soon goes awry. But what was fun is the nest that illustrator John Manders came up with. It's elevated, with a welcome mat, a handy ramp, plump pillows to sit on, a fan placed thoughtfully nearby, and cheery lights strung overhead.

Of course, you wouldn't put a real chicken in this nest. Within a minute she would poop on the pillow, and there goes your perfect nest.

But I wish we could find some compromise between crowded cages in airless, sunless buildings, and Manders's designer nest—some way to keep the hens safe, keep their eggs affordable, yet let them enjoy the sun for a bit, or snag a grasshopper or two. The more I know about eggs, the more I consider them a perfectly packaged miracle. It seems we should revere the one who creates this egg and delivers it to us. Unfortunately, we don't. With so many things wrong in the world, sometimes I feel silly worrying about a hen's quality of life, but I can't help it.

Factory farms also raise broilers, which are chickens bred for meat. Until the early 1980s chicken meat in this country came from hens too old to lay eggs productively. But then McDonald's got the idea for the Chicken McNugget, and we went crazy for them. Suddenly the demand could not be met by old hens, so corporations such as ConAgra and Tyson Foods began raising meat chickens in factories. Today more than 99 percent of the chicken in stores or restaurants has been raised in a factory. Our chicken consumption has doubled since 1970. Four companies now control more than 50 percent of the chicken market.

Fifty years ago chicken was more expensive than beef, but now it's the cheapest meat you can buy.[15]

CAFOs have changed the relationships between farmers, animals, and food companies. In the days of Auntie Em's little brood of peeping chicks in *The Wizard of Oz*, farmers owned the chickens and made all the decisions. That's all changed now, because the big poultry companies own the chicks and make all the decisions. According to Eric Schlosser, author of *Fast Food Nation*, Tyson supplies day-old chicks to farmers, and the chicken farmer provides the land, fuel, labor, and chicken houses, each of which cost about $150,000. Tyson tells the farmer what to feed and how much, and then sets the price for the chickens when they reach market weight thirty-seven days later.[16] Author George Pyle said it well: "The agribusiness giants do not farm the land. They farm the farmers."[17]

The chickens have been bred to gain weight quickly, so instead of taking a few months to gain three pounds, they gain twice that much in half the time and are butchered at four to five weeks of age. Their legs often cannot support their weight. One study found that 90 percent of broilers had detectable leg problems and 26 percent had chronic pain because of bone disease. They also develop heart problems.[18]

The chickens are crammed thirty thousand to a building that is five hundred feet long and forty-five feet wide. Though they are not kept in individual cages, they have only ninety-six square inches in which to move. That's the size of a sheet of eight-and-a-half-by-eleven-inch paper. They're fed arsenic to make them grow faster.

As Roger Caras wrote, "[Chickens] are, unquestionably, one of man's most valuable and readily available sources of food. . . . Yet immeasurably more care is lavished on chickens when they are dead than when they are alive. It is the ultimate separation of man and his deeds, a total indifference to the well-being of animals on which we are so dependent for our well-being."[19]

••• ••• •••

Whether you call them pigs or hogs or swine or Babe, these stout pink or brown animals are smart, sensitive, and they love beer. Sy Montgomery raised a pig named Christopher Hogwood, who loved beer—Rolling Rock, Corona, you name it. Christopher came to love beer so much that if he saw anyone even holding a bottle, "he would chase them until they surrendered and let him suck it dry."

No beer for hogs in confinement, I'm afraid. No living outside, either. You can drive across a major hog-producing state like Iowa and never see a hog. Ninety-five percent of the pigs raised in this country are raised in long, hanger-type buildings from farrow to finish, or as the industry likes to say, "from squeal to meal."

Pregnant sows are kept in individual crates like the one I saw at the state fair. The hogs stand on concrete floors with open slats, so their manure can drop down into pits below. Gases coming off the manure are pulled off the pits by fans and vented outside, but employees wear masks to protect themselves.[20] If a facility's ventilation system broke down for any length of time, pigs would start dying. The pits are emptied periodically, and the manure is either put in large lagoons or spread on nearby fields.

Piglets live with the sow, but not really, since she's restrained in the crate so she won't crush her babies, then are weaned at three weeks and moved into a finishing building, where they're kept in crowded pens, They live there for three or four months until they reach 250 pounds or so.

The animals are given no bedding material because it would interfere with the pits. Sows in stalls bite the bars, chew the air, shake their heads, and nose the empty feed trough. Hogs in confinement experience respiratory problems because of the ammonia and dust in their environment. In addition to toxic fumes, some swine buildings contain bacteria, yeast, and molds at a level more than one thousand times higher than recorded in normal air. The hogs' immune systems are so damaged that they are very susceptible to infections.[21]

Pigs have ulcers on their bodies from rubbing against crates and often come down with foot and leg problems. According to hog industry reports, 70 percent of confined hogs suffer foot and leg infections, skin mange, and chronic respiratory diseases.[22] The confined hogs also bite one another's tails. As a New York hog farmer said, "People think that the pigs are having a problem so they cut off their tails. They disregard the fact that the animals are overcrowded in a tiny pen and that's why they are biting each other."[23] The tails aren't cut entirely off, however; a short stub is left, hopefully tender enough that the pig won't stand still when another pig starts munching on it.

In 1950 two million U.S. hog farms raised 80 million pigs per year. In 2005 only 4 percent of those farms remained, about seventy-five thousand, and they raised 100 million pigs per year.[24] Thanks to a handy USDA table, I learned that of the entire 2005 U.S. inventory of pigs, 89 percent lived on operations of more than 1,000 pigs. Fifty-three percent of the hogs lived in CAFOs of 5,000 or more animals.[25]

•••   •••   •••

Perhaps because of their size, beef cattle are still raised outside. The calves are usually born on small or conventional farms, and if they're lucky, they spend six months with their mother before being weaned. Then they are loaded onto trucks and shipped hundreds of miles to massive feedlots, most of them in Colorado, Kansas, Nebraska, and Texas. According to Michael Pollan, "A feedlot is very much a premodern city . . . teeming and filthy and stinking, with open sewers, unpaved roads, and choking air rendered visible by dust."[26]

I ran back to my USDA 2005 livestock table. Of the inventory of cattle and calves, 77 percent live in feedlots of one hundred or more cattle, and almost 30 percent are in feedlots of more than one thousand. While the USDA's table's highest category is "1000+ head," many of the feedlots are much, much larger. Some contain up to one hundred thousand cattle. Witnesses have referred to a sense of confusion as they near these feedlots, for the earth seems to be moving. Only when they get closer do they realize what they thought was black soil is really the backs of black steers.

As Eric Schlosser writes in *Chew on This*: "These cattle don't wander the prairie, eating fresh grass. During the three months before slaughter, they eat special grain dumped into long concrete troughs that look like highway dividers. The grain is designed to fatten the cattle quickly, aided by growth hormones that have been implanted beneath their skin."[27]

Feedlots are models of efficiency. Steers used to take four or five years to reach slaughter weight, but in the 1950s that number dropped to two or three years. Thanks to modern agricultural methods, a steer can now be finished in fourteen to sixteen months.

In a typical feedlot a cow's diet is roughly 95 percent grain. According to Schlosser, a steer will consume three thousand pounds of grain in order to gain four hundred pounds. (Each steer produces fifty pounds of urine and manure every day, a fact that we'll be discussing more later.) A diet this high in grain lowers the pH in the animal's rumen. Antibiotics are necessary to keep the liver functioning long enough for the animal to reach slaughter weight. It's been estimated that 70 percent of the antibiotics dispensed in this country are given to animals.[28]

Feedlot cattle come from many conventional farming cow/calf operations, where pregnant cows give birth, raise those calves for a number of months, then the calves are sold to feedlots. These are animals bred specifically for meat. Dairy calves that are not needed on the dairies also end up at feedlots. The feedlots fatten both male and female cattle, although not usually together.

Male calves are castrated, but because it isn't cost effective to perform little hysterectomies on the heifers, feedlots use hormones to control the heifers' estrous cycles.

Before they began this practice, when feedlot heifers regularly went through their reproductive cycle there were lots of problems. When cycling, a heifer's natural tendency is to ride other animals, which stirs up dust, and bruises the animals being ridden. Once feedlots put the heifers on birth control, there was less riding, less carcass bruising, and the heifers settled down quicker, were more content, and more relaxed.[29]

Dairy farming has followed the same path as the cattle industry—overcrowding, hormone use, and antibiotic use. Dairies have supersized as well. The average herd size has increased from 100 cows to 850.[30] This is small, however, compared to the really big dairies, milking 10,000 to 18,000 cows a day.[31] A Cornell University study predicts we'll go from 105,000 dairies in 2000 to 16,000 by 2020, yet the total milk production and number of cows per dairy will increase.

Cows are usually milked twice a day, so they need to be kept fairly close to the milking parlor. Many never leave the barn or loafing shed, and some dairies keep each cow confined for most of the year in a tie stall, where she lives, eats, and is milked. Of the USDA 2005 inventory of milk cows, 44 percent were on farms with more than five hundred head.

Dairy cows are fed the same grain-based diet as beef cattle. A display in the dairy barn at the Minnesota State Fair announced that a cow that is fed only pasture will produce fifty glasses of milk per day, but a cow on a mixed diet of grain and hay will produce one hundred glasses a day. In addition to the rumen problems associated with a grain-based diet, dairy cows suffer from additional problems related to being milked so heavily. Since the mid-1990s, dairy cows have been given rBST, which is a genetically engineered version of the naturally occurring hormone bovine somatotropin, or BST, to increase milk production. In 1967 a cow produced nine thousand pounds of milk per year, but by 2002 she produced a whopping sixteen thousand pounds a year.[32]

Whether or not you believe the studies claiming these hormones represent risks to human health when the hormones pass through the milk into our bodies, at the very least they make life difficult for the cows. The natural life of a dairy cow is about twenty years, but cows given hormones for super-production burn out in five years and are sold for meat. With such huge udders, cows easily suffer from mastitis, a common disease that leads to increased use of antibiotics. Some dairies can't be bothered with treating ill animals, however, so they just ship them off to the livestock market to once again be sold for meat. The issue isn't that dairy cows become meat. The issue is that their bodies are pushed to the limits by factory dairying.

With meat chickens, beef steers, hogs, and sheep, the animals reproduce to make more animals, since that's the product we sell. But on a dairy, cows give birth not for the calves, but for the milk the cow's body produces to feed the calf. Some dairies sell their calves to local farmers to raise, which is how Melissa and I acquired our steer. Others put some of the calves into small pens—in our area they are little white igloos with a tiny fenced area attached, about as long as the calf itself—and raise them for sixteen weeks as veal.

I've read disturbing accounts, however, of dairies that load the very young calves into trucks and ship them to a livestock market. The cow goes through pregnancy and birth without ever seeing or nursing her calf. I've also read of a dairy tossing aside its newborn calves and letting them die.[33] I don't want to believe this is true. I want to believe a farmer would not be this cruel and unfeeling to bring an animal into the world only to let it die because it's too much trouble to bottle-feed it, or to find someone else who will.

···   ···   ···

Sheep might be the least industrialized of all the livestock animals, and I'm not sure why. Perhaps because lamb's share of the meat market is too small to attract much attention. Most of the U.S. lamb is raised in feedlots in California, Colorado, Texas, and Wyoming. These feedlots represent about 2 percent of the total number of U.S. lamb producers, but raise more than 50 percent of the lamb and mutton sold.[34] These guys are *big.*

Most lambs are born on farms and ranches, then when they're about sixty pounds, they're sold as "feeders" to the big guys to finish. The feedlot owner switches the lambs from mostly roughage—pasture or hay—to a high-concentrate diet of grain. Animals in feedlots have nothing to do but stand around and wait for their next meal. We visited a lamb feedlot in southeastern Minnesota, and the only word I can use to describe it is *dusty.* There was no vegetation on the ground, the sheep having long since eaten it. It was a sea of white, wooly backs.

···   ···   ···

Does it bother chickens and cattle and hogs to be packed together in factories and feedlots? I remember reading somewhere that a cattleman with a massive feedlot was overheard to say that his cattle were perfectly content in their feedlot and didn't feel any lack because of it. Someone then urged him to open the gate, let the cattle decide between a crowded feedlot and the open range, and see what would happen. The man declined.

Tom Frantzen of Iowa raised hogs in confinement for fourteen years and became increasingly frustrated because the system "treated animals as machines, manure as waste, and farmers as barnyard janitors." He and his family visited Sweden, saw there was an alternative to hog factories, and made the change, replacing buildings and concrete floors with pastures and Swedish-style, open hoop-shaped shelters with straw floors. Frantzen described what happened the day he moved his hogs from confinement into the new pasture-and-straw-based system: "They ran around all day long, and they must have run around all night long, too, because when I went out to the building the next morning I will never forget what I found. I peeked into the hoop house to see 180 pigs in one massive straw nest—snoring. I laughed until I cried. Their stress was gone, and so was mine."[35]

I love this image of all those previously confined hogs piled together, touching, snoring in satisfaction after running their butts off all day. That's how an animal should live, and it makes me want to run out and buy myself some pigs.

There are a few rays of hope. The gestation crates will be illegal in the entire European Union after 2013.[36] Oregon, Arizona, and Florida have implemented a similar ban.[37] In March 2007 Burger King announced it would begin buying eggs and pork from suppliers that don't confine their animals in cages and crates. The company's initial goals were to purchase 2 percent of their eggs and 10 percent of the pork from such suppliers, and they intend to increase the percentages as more farmers shift to non-confinement methods.[38]

Two months earlier, perhaps seeing the writing on the wall, Smithfield Foods, which raises sows at 187 locations in eight states and produces 27 percent of the country's pork, said it would begin replacing the individual sow crates with pens where the sows can move around and be housed in groups.[39] These are small, encouraging steps, but it's hard to predict how long it will take to affect the entire industry, or if it even will.

When I become discouraged about changing how I eat meat, or confused by conflicting claims of researchers and agribusiness, I conjure up the image of Frantzen's pile of sleeping pigs and remember my one constant truth: it's about the animals. Because animals matter, it's my responsibility, as a meat eater, to ensure they actually have some quality of life.

Once the animals have paid a big chunk of the externalities so that people can buy cheap meat from factories, then it's the planet's turn, so hold your breath for one more dunking in the dip tank.

# That's One
# Heck of a Hoofprint

••• ••• •••••• ••• •••

MOST PEOPLE CAN'T pick up a magazine or newspaper, or listen to public radio, without hearing about global warming, about reducing our carbon footprint on the earth, about going a little easier on the planet. Catalogs and magazines and organizations have sprung up eagerly to help us become greener consumers.

As environmentalists have been trying to pound into our heads for so many years, modern agriculture hasn't been kind to Mother Nature. And since we've been letting modern agriculture feed us like helpless baby birds, we're responsible for the externalities streaming from factory farms.

I'm sorry to report I'm not the greenest of people. While I both read Al Gore's *An Inconvenient Truth* and watched the movie of the same name, some days the whole global warming thing feels too huge to ever overcome. I do my best to recycle, but I've been known to toss the tuna can into the trash with only the tiniest twinge of guilt. Living out in the country, we must load our recyclables into the car, take them into town, and dump them in the correct bin. Some days it's too much for me, and I'm tempted to throw two months' worth of catalogs (about seven full grocery bags) directly into our dumpster. When we had goats, most of our vegetable waste went straight into their mouths, but now that we don't, the compost pile is just too darned far away. No, my environmental philosophy is greener than my actual practice.

Perhaps that's why I approached looking closer at the environmental impacts of livestock farming with some trepidation, and lots of exhaustion. Yes, I'm a sustainable farmer, and I do care about the earth, but some days I'm not all that consistent about it.

I'm pretty sure I'm not alone in this struggle. The other day I walked by a *towering* black SUV parked in town, with a "Go Organic" bumper sticker on the back. It made me smile. At least the driver's trying, which some days is all we can expect from one another.

As a farmer, I try to avoid all of those overly romantic terms that create rosy portraits of farmers as altruistic "stewards of the land" or people "living off the land." I think it's important to put agricultural land to agricultural use rather than turning productive land into huge fields of wildflowers or forty-acre playgrounds for two horses. While legally we own the land, we're really just taking care of it until the next guy takes over. Melissa and I believe it's our responsibility to leave the land in just as good a shape, if not better, as when we started. CAFOs feel no such responsibility and severely impact the water, air, and soil.

Animal manure never used to be a problem when lots of farmers raised a few animals. A farmer with one hundred cows or hogs would either let the animals distribute their own manure by walking around the pastures, or if the animals had access to the barn, the farmer periodically cleaned out the barn and gathered the manure. He'd fill up his manure spreader (basically a long box with a spinning mechanism along the back end), hook the spreader up to the tractor, rumble out to his cropland, and spread the manure. A spreader spitting out big clods of poop is an impressive sight, but steering clear of the spreader is obviously a good idea, as is closing your car window if you happen to be driving by.

The soil microbes immediately begin to break down the manure, and rain liquefies some of it, so it soaks into the soil, where the roots of plants—corn, oats, alfalfa, wheat, or grass—reach out and suck up the nutrients. The plants use those nutrients to grow big and strong and produce pasture or a healthy crop of grain—which is fed either to meat animals or to us—and pasture. The animals produce more waste, which is spread on the fields to help grow more crops or pasture. It's a pretty nifty system, actually.

Then corporations started supersizing farms, and suddenly manure became a problem. How do you handle the manure of five hundred thousand hogs or one hundred thousand cattle? At a Smithfield plant in Utah that houses five hundred thousand hogs, more fecal matter gets produced in one year than is created by all the inhabitants of Manhattan.[40]

One sow and her approximately twenty piglets born in a year will produce 1.9 tons of manure, enough to fill the bed of a standard pickup truck.[41] If one hog operation has twenty thousand hogs, it's generating enough manure to fill twenty thousand pickups. Here's a manure disposal idea: since pickup trucks have become increasingly popular with urban dwellers but seem to be rarely used to transport stuff, why not fill these empty beds with the manure our meat produces?

Okay, probably not. Instead, the corporations build huge lagoons, fill them with manure, and then spread the liquid manure over fields. But suddenly that neat little closed system doesn't work so well, because they're putting too much fertilizer out there. Soil can only absorb so much.

The excess nitrogen that the soil and crops can't absorb hangs around looking for a place to go, and rain is the perfect transportation system, picking up the nitrogen and delivering it down the rivulets, which head for the streams, which head for rivers, lakes, and oceans. According to the U.S. Environmental Protection Agency, the twenty-two states that list specific categories of agricultural pollution concluded that animal wastes pollute about thirty-five thousand of the river miles they assessed.[42]

Also, the lagoons themselves have been known to leak. According to a U.S. Senate Committee on Agriculture, during 1992 twenty hog manure spills in Iowa, Minnesota, and Missouri killed more than 55,000 fish. By 1996 the number of spills had doubled, killing off 670,000 fish. Between 1995 and 1998 there were over 1,000 lagoon spills or leaking incidents at feedlots in ten states, and two hundred manure-related fish kills.[43] In 2002 Nebraska's Department of Environmental Quality tested one-third of the state's more than 16,000 miles of rivers and found 71 percent were polluted.[44]

Up to half of factory manure nutrients get washed into streams or filter down into groundwater, then into aquifers, then into people's wells. High nitrate levels in wells near feedlots have been linked to greater risks of miscarriage. Nitrate contamination can cause blue baby syndrome, infant poisoning in which the blood's ability to carry oxygen is severely impaired.[45]

In the spring of 2000 in Walkerton, Ontario, more than one thousand people got sick, and four died, from E. coli because the municipal water system had been contaminated by feedlot runoff.[46] Sussex County, Delaware, produces 232 million chickens every year, but a University of Delaware study found the county has enough land to cope with the manure from only one-quarter of those chickens.[47] During the 1990s one-third of the wells in this area exceeded EPA standards for nitrates.[48]

Hormones fed to animals end up in rivers and streams. Fish exposed to feedlot effluent end up with their reproductive systems very messed up. Also, excess nutrients stimulate excessive algae growth. After the algae dies, the decomposition process removes oxygen from the water and fish die. In July 2003 a dead

zone stretched for one hundred miles down the center of Chesapeake Bay.[49]

This is nothing compared to the dead zone in the Gulf of
Mexico that ranges in size from five thousand to eight thousand
square miles, about the size of New Jersey. The Mississippi and
Atchafalaya Rivers flow into the gulf, and these two rivers drain
about 40 percent of all U.S. land. The National Oceanic and At-
mospheric Administration has identified the culprit as the excess
nutrients from agricultural fertilizers that run off into the two
river basins. "Fish, shrimp, and all other marine organisms that
require oxygen to survive either flee the zone or die."[50]

When raw manure is exposed to air, the nitrogen can turn
into gaseous ammonia and doesn't smell good. When you have
high quantities of manure concentrated in one place, the smell
shifts from a quaint, country smell to significant air pollution.
The best way to experience these odors, short of some sort of
scratch-'n-sniff insert in this book, is through the words of people
who've breathed them. A Kansas State University professor
wrote: "There is nothing like a hundred thousand head of hogs
in a containment facility on a hot July day. It'll bring you to
your knees and put tears in your eyes."[51]

University of North Carolina researchers found that people living near large hog farms suffer significantly higher levels of upper
respiratory and gastrointestinal ailments than people living near
large cattle farms or in non-livestock areas. An Iowa study found
that people living near large hog facilities came down with the
same respiratory problems as did those working in hog confinement operations.

North Carolina's Duke University medical center discovered
that people exposed to the swine odors suffered from "significantly
more tension, more depression, more anger, less vigor, more fatigue, and more confusion than control subjects."[52] A resident of
western Kentucky gives what she calls the "Tour de Stench," a

drive through a rural area loaded with chicken farms, so that legislators and others can experience the impacts on the environment. One stop on the tour is Bernadine Edwards's house, whose neighbors contracted with Tyson Foods in 1997 to operate a chicken factory on their property.

There are now ninety-two chicken buildings within a three-mile radius of Edwards's home, and the neighbor's operation across the road has grown to sixteen buildings containing nearly half a million birds. "The fecal dust, chemicals, and smell from that place keep us indoors most days," she says. "I have to keep my windows shut, and the house gets coated with grime; a lot of days it's crawling with flies."[53]

We, as consumers, are paying Tyson Foods to raise chickens as cheaply as it can. We are not paying for the health costs associated with the raising of those chickens. We are not compensating Bernadine Edwards for not being able to breathe when she is standing outside her own home. If meat producers were forced to reduce the toxic gases coming from their factories, the price of meat would go up, thereby forcing the meat consumers to pay for the externalities instead of the unfortunate neighbors of the factories.

Exporting our factory system to the rest of the world is having the same negative effects in other places as it is here in the United States. In 1998 Smithfield proclaimed it was going to turn Poland into "the Iowa of Europe" and began building factory hog farms. Its local subsidiary now runs twenty-nine farms and raises 1.3 million hogs per year. One of those farms, with 12,000 hogs, is near Wiekowice, a small town of seven hundred people. The factory's waste disposal system was built near an elementary school, and kids soon began vomiting and fainting. The company moved the site farther away, near a lake, and now swimmers get eye infections when they swim there.[54]

As the U.N. Food and Agricultural Organization's Pierre Gerber wrote: "While farmers with five pigs can have a well managed, well developed, closed-loop recycling system where they use manure to fertilize their crops, . . . farmers with 500 or more pigs can no longer follow these ancient practices."[55]

Until we started the farm, I thought of soil as being another word for dirt, so I didn't pay much attention to the idea of soil and what it actually is. Soil is alive, packed full of little living microbes whose job it is to break down dead matter, thereby making that matter's nutrients available for plants to suck up through their roots. The microbes need oxygen to breathe, and they give off carbon dioxide just like we do. Soil is also made up of the nutrient-rich worm castings (a fancy word for worm poop).

Modern farming does nasty stuff to this living, breathing world beneath our feet. It disturbs massive tracts of land, plowing it up in order to plant crops. Every time you expose the soil to the elements, you start losing it. More than two billion tons of soil are lost annually through wind and soil erosion thanks to modern agricultural practices.[56] The soil that's left contains fewer nutrients, so the farmers apply more and more chemical fertilizers, some of which run off into our water supply and contaminate it. Also, farmers apply anhydrous nitrogen as fertilizer, and this kills the soil's microbes.

Concentrating large groups of animals, or running a tractor repeatedly over a piece of land, compacts the soil. This hardens the top layer so much that oxygen can no longer penetrate the surface and carbon dioxide (given off by the microbes) can't escape. Not enough oxygen and too much carbon dioxide means the microbes suffocate. The soil dies.

Large-scale crop farming, the products of which 70 percent are fed to livestock, applies chemical pesticides to rid crops of insects. We're using over thirty-three times more pesticides than we used fifty years ago.[57] In what's called a pesticide treadmill, the insects become resistant, so the growers apply more per acre. When pesticides kill off an entire species in the area, everything gets off balance.

Factory farms are hard on the animals, water, air, soil, and neighbors. A research and advocacy group called Food and Water Watch wants you to know where the factory farms are located. Visiting http://www.factoryfarmmap.org shows you the concentration of factory farms, by product, across the country. It doesn't pinpoint the farms exactly, but just the statewide totals.

There is some good news. Sometimes the EPA does level fines, thereby making the corporate farms pay for some of their externalities. In 2001 the EPA compelled five hog operations in two Oklahoma counties to provide area residents with safe drinking water, since nitrates from the hog operations had contaminated both the aquifer and area drinking-water wells.

A lawsuit was brought against Tyson in Madisonville, Kentucky, but Tyson said that because it didn't own the factories, but only contracted with the growers, it wasn't responsible. A 2003 federal court rejected the argument, ruling that because Tyson controlled every step of the chicken-raising process, the company was indeed responsible. A five-hundred-thousand-dollar settlement was reached in 2005, requiring Tyson to study the problem, plant trees, and reduce odors.[58]

Both conventional farmers and CAFOs have figured out that their manure problems might be turned into energy solutions. Manure is a great source of methane gas, which can be used to power a generator. Blue Spruce Farm is a Vermont dairy that is doing that very thing, using a methane digester to extract methane from the manure of two thousand cows. By producing electricity and selling some back to the local power company, the farm has reduced its net power costs to zero. Not only is the farm producing energy, but it's also removing about 90 percent of the smell from the manure. The farmers use the by-product, steril- ized manure, as a bedding for the cows instead of sawdust, saving the dairy as much as one hundred thousand dollars annually, not to mention a few trees.[59]

Hog farmers are beginning to consider similar ideas but haven't progressed much beyond the experimental stage. A pork produc- tion network in Illinois is working with the EPA to study the feasi- bility of producing electricity from methane. A Smithfield subsidiary in North Carolina covered about 20 percent of a ma- nure lagoon with black plastic tarp to capture the methane gas that rises off the pond as the manure decomposes.[60] North Carolina is the second-largest hog producer in the United States, with twenty-three hundred farms raising more than nine million hogs, so if those farms could capture and convert the methane, they could produce enough electricity to power about fifty thousand homes. However, covering the lagoons may not be as effective as fully treat- ing the waste, and farmers aren't likely to invest in the necessary equipment unless there's a significant cost savings involved.

Energy can be produced from an amazing range of material, including hog manure, but whether it's actually done depends on economics. When I was in graduate school, my master's degree project was to study the economic feasibility of cattails as an al- ternative source of energy for Minnesota. (Don't laugh. Biomass was big back then.) While the process of converting either the cattail stalks or the roots was scientifically feasible, the fuel cre- ated would have been too expensive. This is why you don't see cattail fuel at your local gas station, and why corporations won't invest in manure-to-power systems unless those systems will save them money. Not to keep hammering on the same nail, but if CAFOs were forced to pay for the externalities they create, then converting manure to power might look like a smart investment to them.

Livestock emit about 18 percent of the world's annual quantity of methane, one of the bad boys responsible for global warming.[61] They produce this methane as part of their digestion process, and most of it comes out in burps. But Dr. Winfried Drochner, a German scientist, is developing a large pill for livestock (called a bolus) that's made of "microbially active substances" that would remain in a cow's stomach for a few months, slowly dissolving and reducing methane emissions.[62] Another researcher is recommending diet changes, among them feeding livestock a weed called bird's-foot trefoil. Not to sound smug, but our pasture is full of bird's-foot trefoil, so I guess our sheep aren't burping out as much methane as other sheep. And not to get picky, but anything our sheep will eat isn't a weed—it's food.

These research experiments are steps in the right direction, but they don't change an animal's life inside a CAFO, and realistically, they won't have any large-scale impact on the environment for years. Besides, while we've relied on technology to solve so many of our agricultural problems, technology has also created its share of problems, especially for livestock animals. Instead of looking to technology for the solution, *we* can solve the animal welfare and environmental issues surrounding meat by getting into grass.

Part Four

# As Green as It Gets

Good food . . . comes from good farming.

—WENDELL BERRY

My dad isn't what you'd call a "grass man." He's hated yard work for as long as I can remember, and would much rather be putting together a model airplane, looking through motorcycle catalogs, or selling brats for the Shriners booth at summer festivals. It's no surprise that he and my stepmother live in a townhouse where someone else mows the lawn.

My stepfather, on the other hand, is very serious about his grass. He mows in both directions for a fluffy lawn. He trims, weeds, and waters until you'd swear you were walking on carpeting. If he were to suddenly need emergency surgery, he'd first insist that my mom drive him home so that he could put the lawn in order before going under the knife.

For most of us, our experience with grass is limited to lawns. We struggle to grow them or cut them or eliminate their weeds. But for the aware carnivore, the significance of grass reaches well beyond the edges of your lawn, basically because it's green.

Green used to be the mild-mannered color nestled between blue and yellow on the color wheel, but now it's recycling and saving energy and eating locally and driving hybrid cars and being responsible. If you want to trace green's journey from a lowly color to a global powerhouse, all you need to do is head outside and find a piece of ground that isn't concrete, blacktop, sand, or rock, then look down at your feet.

There it is, soft and thick, or sparse and prickly. In the context of farming, grass is actually any green plant, and it's the basis for the type of farming that used to dominate the U.S. agricultural scene and is now making a comeback: sustainable, pasture-based livestock farms. As we start paying more attention to the idea of grass and pasture, where should we fall in the continuum between my father the Grass Phobe and my stepfather the Grass Guru? In a dazzling display of family and parental peacekeeping skills, I say we should come down squarely halfway between them. While we need to pay more attention to grass and what it means to us, we also don't need to obsess about it either.

Grass-fed. Pasture-raised. These terms might be tossed about interchangeably by many, and that's okay, since they lead to the same conclusion: If a meat eater is going to change how she eats meat, she'll need to accept that not only are animals affected by what they eat, but *we* are affected by what *animals* eat. If we don't want animals raised on grain in factories, we'll want animals raised outside on grass.

# Sustainable Is More
# Than a Buzzword

••• ••• •••••• ••• •••

*SUSTAINABLE* HAS BECOME a trendy word, tossed about willy-nilly by people who have no idea what sustainable really means, which can be terribly irksome to those of us who've been practicing it for years. The example that really elevated my blood pressure was the 2007 *Newsweek* article about fashion designers proudly announcing new lines of clothing made from Ingeo, which is a fabric made from corn.[1]

While this Ingeo material is "thin and comfortable," and "doesn't stretch or rip," designers are also using the corn fabric because "corn is sustainable." What? Corn? Sustainable? Michael Pollan wrote an entire book centered on corn and how it is totally *not* sustainable.[2] Growing corn in this country requires huge amounts of fossil fuel to run the tractors and produce and apply the chemical fertilizers, herbicides, and insecticides. Gigantic fields of corn are planted, horizon to horizon, with little concern for wind erosion, chemical runoff into the water supply, or the effect on the wildlife of applying poisons to the crops. Renewable? Yes. Sustainable? No. If we are going to start calling industrial corn sustainable, then we might as well say that petroleum is a re-newable resource if you're willing to wait long enough.

This is why it's so important for you, as a conscious carnivore, to understand what a sustainable farm looks like and how it might operate, since I fear there are some who would jump on the sustainable bandwagon and proclaim to be something they're not.

According to Webster's dictionary, *sustainable* is "a method of harvesting or using a resource so that the resource is not depleted or permanently damaged." When we began farming, the working definition of sustainability was a three-legged stool: economic vi-ability (the farmer needs to make a profit); environmental re-sponsibility (the farming practices should enhance and protect the environment rather than deplete it); and quality of life (for both the farmer and the farmer's livestock). You need all three legs or the stool will fall over.

A sustainable farm may look and operate like a pre–World War II farm, before the USDA and chemical companies and large tractors created modern agriculture. A sustainable farm pays attention to what animals need not just to stay alive but to thrive, to live as close to a natural life as possible, and still recognize that farming is a business. Sustainable farming isn't a hobby; no one in their right mind would work this hard on a hobby.

Sustainable farming returns to an idea that worked for thou-sands of years: kicking the animals out of the barn and putting them out into the pasture. Making them actually walk around, harvesting the grass and clover and dandelions, letting them spread their own manure. Letting them roll in the mud or root in the ground. Giving them the bedding materials and food and space that best fit their lives.

The desire to raise animals naturally cuts across religious and political barriers. Robert Hutchins calls himself a Christian fundamentalist sustainable farmer. "We raise our cattle the natural way, and feed them only what they were designed to eat. . . . We look at it as honoring God's creation. . . . On factory farms [humans] think we know better than God about how to raise these animals. That's simply not true."[3]

Sustainable farmers are comfortable with uncertainty. I heard a speaker the other day contrast the skills of conventional farmers with those of farmers using a pasture-based system. Conventional farmers like certainty; they like knowing that if they feed their animals so many pounds of corn a day, and so much hay, and maintain a certain regime of hormones, then they can be reasonably certain that their animals will produce a consistent amount of meat.

Pasture-based farmers, on the other hand, are constantly adjusting what they do. They must take everything into account—soil fertility, slope of the land, natural resources available, water—as they design a farming system to best fit their land. The plans for one farm will be different from those of a farm five miles away. Sustainable farmers are always asking themselves: What does my land need? How can I improve it? What's the best way to use it responsibly?

They're watching how quickly the grass is growing. Is the nutritional content of this pasture high enough? Will this pasture bounce back before the animals are scheduled to graze there again? Are noxious weeds crowding out the edible plants? Are the animals carrying a heavy worm load in their intestines? To be a pasture-based farmer is to be a person willing to make changes. If you ask Melissa which pasture the sheep will be grazing next week, she may not have an answer, since it depends on the mix of plants in each pasture and which is growing back the fastest.

Although sustainable farms may look very different from one another, they all follow these basic principles:

- Use animal manure and crop rotation to fertilize the soil instead of using chemicals.
- Manage weeds and insects using minimal insecticides or herbicides.
- Put ruminants (cud-chewing animals, such as cattle, sheep, and goats) out on pasture, using rotational grazing to most effectively harvest the grass.
- Don't use hormones to encourage growth.
- Don't use antibiotics unless necessary. If a farmer treats an animal with antibiotics, she will not sell the meat to customers as antibiotic-free meat. At the same time, she will not withhold life-saving drugs just to keep the animals free of antibiotics.

We need to avoid antibiotic hysteria, labeling farmers as bad if they use them. We *all* use them, because they are important tools for saving an animal's life. If you get a serious infection and a dose of antibiotics will help cure you, you should take the antibiotics. If one of our animals becomes ill and a dose of antibiotics will cure that animal, we use the antibiotics. But there is a huge difference between treating a sick animal with antibiotics and using antibiotics to keep an animal healthy in unhealthy conditions.

Sustainable agriculture leaves a smaller hoofprint. The water supply is safer, because the farms are supporting fewer animals, so less manure runs off into streams. Some runoff may still occur, but not to the scale of a factory farm. Farmers may compost the manure they've cleaned out of a barn or feedlot. They may spread it on their fields. Pasture-based systems usually don't have manure-handling issues, since the animals walk around and deposit the manure themselves.

Our sheep are rarely in the barn, so their manure doesn't really accumulate. What they leave behind just sits there composting.

After our first few years of farming, the barn floor was basically a three-inch layer of rich, loamy, composted soil. I knew we had something good going when my mom, the gardener, began stealing our barn floor.

Small farms, sustainable or conventional, don't smell that bad. Some conventional feedlots can emit a nice little stink, but it's a fairly small stink, one you won't notice unless you're driving by. About a mile to the west of our farm, there's a small farmer who agitates his manure lagoon about twice a month to incorporate more oxygen for faster decomposition. On those days, the smell drifts our way. But it only lasts a day or two, and any person who moves into an agricultural area needs to accept the fact that there will be smells. But the fewer the animals, and the more spread out they are, the less the stink.

Sustainable farmers avoid using herbicides to control weeds but look to more natural methods, such as planting cover crops, mechanical control of weeds, or mulching. Sustainable farmers avoid chemicals because they recognize that soil is everything. Before we bought our land, it had been farmed extensively with corn and soybeans, so the soil's nutrients had been grossly depleted. The topsoil was laughable, having long since eroded down the hill into a small creek valley. There wasn't an earthworm to be seen, since earthworms can't survive in compacted soil poisoned with chemicals.

We don't disturb the soil. If we need to reseed the pasture, we rent a no-till drill, which plants seeds in the ground without disturbing the soil. We don't use insecticides unless a wasp has built a nest over our front door. We don't use herbicides except to control weeds around our grapevines. We don't compress the soil, since our tractor only passes over the pastures maybe once a year as Melissa mows.

Twelve years later, the roots of our perennial grasses hold the soil in place, so it no longer erodes. The earthworms are everywhere;

their tunnels have aerated the soil and their castings have fertilized it. I know they're everywhere because I've heard them. One
evening at dusk after a rainstorm, I walked across the lawn and
heard the weirdest little sucking noises, almost as if the ground
was breathing. The sounds came from all around me, twenty feet
in every direction. A little freaked, I brought Melissa out to hear
the sounds, because she and Mother Nature have been buddies
since Melissa was a kid. "Oh, those are the worms," she said after
I took a few steps to set off the soft, wet popping sounds all
around us. "When they're crawling around on the surface, they
can hear or feel you approach. They don't want to be eaten, so
they scoot back down into their tunnels. The sound you hear is
the worms making their escape."

We've restored some diversity to the farm. Pheasants and Hun-
garian partridge and meadowlarks nest in the pasture. Bluebirds
show up every spring and make babies. Spring peepers, or little
frogs, set up a rousing chorus every night.

I chose not to have children, so that's not a legacy I can leave.
But taking fifty-three acres and letting Mother Nature work the
way she's supposed to work—keeping the air clean and fresh; ensuring clean water for animals, fish, and people; and bringing the
soil back to life—feels pretty darned good.

# Grass Farming
# as Aerobic Exercise

··· ··· ······ ··· ···

WHEN SHEEP, GOATS, or hogs are raised in pens, they are crowded in tightly enough that it's not too hard to wade into the bunch and snag the animal you want or run them through a sorting gate. In cattle feedlots an employee on horseback cuts out a sick steer and moves it into a hospital pen. The animals are all in the same place, accessible, and fairly under control, which appeals to many farmers. There are some days when this sounds pretty good to a pasture-based farmer as well. Imagine if a stressed-out teacher could corral all the students and keep them in a small pen at the center of the room. Think control. Think how much calmer her day would be.

Is living on a sustainable farm easier for an animal than living in a factory? Absolutely. But it might be a little more difficult for the farmer, since along with balancing many scientific factors—growth of the plants, nutritional requirements of the animals during different stages of their lives, weather problems—sustainable farmers must also deal with catching and treating a sick animal on pasture.

Sheep can be handled only if you can get your hands on the little buggers. Our sheep aren't penned in a barn, where they're easy to catch by chasing them into a corner and grabbing them. Instead, they're out on pasture, grazing. They aren't pets and don't come when called, so we must be creative in our sheep-catching methods.

The first year we had sheep I was stunned by the animals' speed, grace, leaping, and general ability to evade me. I learned that a cornered, frightened ewe will go right through, or right over, a three-wire electric fence. I learned that a cornered sheep will go right through, or right over, a five-wire electric fence. I finally learned to stop cornering our ewes.

The cheetah is considered the fastest land animal on the planet. It turns out that lambs are actually tiny, fuzzy cheetahs and are impossible to catch. Say you are spry enough to get your hand close to the back end of a running lamb. Just as you lunge, the lamb instinctively drops its hips and all you grab is air, while the lamb scoots off to brag to his friends that he once again eluded the lumbering human.

Our first year with lambs, after we spent an embarrassing amount of time chasing "cheetahs," I finally told Melissa I was no longer going to participate in such a futile activity.

A few weeks later she called to me from the front door, saying she'd seen a limping lamb that we needed to catch and examine. When I reached the door, ready to proclaim I wasn't chasing that lamb, I found her on the front step holding a massive fishing net.

"You're kidding," I said.

"Nope, c'mon. It'll be fun."

The net was two feet long, and the handle extended four feet, which meant we still needed to come within six feet of the fleeing lamb in order to net him. It is humiliating to admit how long it took two healthy, fairly in-shape women to catch a gimpy baby lamb. We finally grew desperate enough that we sort of threw the net at the lamb, and he got tangled up enough that we could at least catch up with the handle.

That's why on some days the idea of putting animals into feedlots actually sounds appealing, since it would make farming less of an aerobic activity.

Our animals not only graze out on pasture, but they're born there as well. During lambing—the big event on a sheep farm when all the ewes give birth—most sheep farmers will put the pregnant ewes that are just about to give birth in small pens, or "jugs." The ewe lives in the jug for a few days so that she and her newborn lambs can bond, then the farmer will start combining family groups into larger pens. Each ewe is fed and watered individually, and to treat a lamb the farmer just has to reach down into the pen and lift the baby out.

The alternative is to lamb out on pasture, which has its challenges. Melissa loves roaming the pasture in May, watching a ewe for signs she's going into labor, then deciding when labor's gone on too long and whether the ewe might need help. One evening during last year's lambing this very situation arose, so Melissa called for reinforcements: me. (I should mention that my idea of a good day on the farm is one where I can remain clean, dry, and free of an animal's bodily fluids.)

To catch this one ewe with birthing problems we had to surround the entire flock with a portable fence, then Melissa chased the ewe in question, finally throwing herself into the middle of the alarmed flock and grabbing the ewe by one back leg. The rest of the sheep scattered, and I watched as the ewe dragged Melissa across the wet pasture. "Could you stop her?" came the polite request, so I belatedly sprang into action and planted myself in front of the ewe to stop her from running. "Thanks," Melissa said, facedown in the wet grass.

After Melissa helped deliver twins, and the ewe cleaned off both lambs and encouraged them to stand and nurse, we left them alone. Once the lambs are at least a few hours old, Melissa then returns to the pasture to "process" them. She approaches the nearest lamb, now dry and alert and fed, who looks up at her in total innocence, and she picks him up. The ewe stomps and snorts and bellows, circling nervously ten feet away. Melissa sits down, puts the lamb in her lap, and does her thing: ear tag for ID, rubber band on the tail to dock it (the tail will eventually atrophy and fall off), iodine on the navel, and a shot of vitamins. Just before she sends the lamb back to its mama, she gives it a kiss on the head. Once she lets that lamb go, the chances of catching it again are not good, and may involve the fishing net.

The sustainable farmer must balance the sheep's needs with those of the pasture. A sheep left to her own devices will roam through a pasture, eating only her favorite green bits, leaving the less tasty stuff to continue growing until it's long and stemmy and really unpalatable. The ewe keeps eating those favorite green stems so close to the ground that her muzzle gets dirty. The plants, now nothing but roots, struggle to survive by pushing up slender new blades of grass, which the ewe promptly chomps off. The tasty stuff dies, and the less palatable stuff takes over the pasture.

Sustainable farmers therefore manage their pastures by using rotational grazing. We set up fencing to keep the animals in an area large enough to contain enough food, but small enough that the animals are forced to feed on *all* the plants, not just the tastiest. After a day or two, the sheep have eaten the grass down to a uniform length, so it's time to move them on before they can harm the plant.

So on they go, leaving behind that spot of pasture to recover. The plants begin to grow again. If there are any parasite eggs in the grass, they will hatch out and die before the sheep can return to ingest them. The manure left behind begins to break down, thanks to insects and weather. We let that piece of land rest for three weeks. By then the sheep need more food, so we move the sheep back into that paddock, and the cycle begins again.

A farm that practices rotational grazing is a quiet farm. There isn't a lot of tractor activity, since you aren't tilling the soil, planting a crop, cultivating, or harvesting using machinery. You're doing all of that with your cattle or sheep. Because we have more land than sheep, sometimes the grass begins to get dangerously long, making it unpalatable to even the least fussy of eaters, so Melissa must fire up the tractor and mow off the grass. But other than this, there's very little for our stalwart Farmall 706 to do in the summer.

Sustainable livestock farmers like to call ourselves grass farmers, believing that our most important product is the grass we grow, and that the sheep and cattle are the best tools for harvesting the grass and converting it into edible energy. We also call ourselves graziers, because we raise grazing animals (not because we ourselves graze).

Remember that three-legged stool called sustainable farming? While two of the legs—economics and the environment—are key, they aren't enough for most of us to keep working this hard. But the third leg—quality of life for the farmer (and the animal)—is why most of us continue to do what we do.

# It's a Chicken's (and Pig's and Sheep's and Steer's and Cow's) Life

... ... ...... ... ...

THE FATE OF animals raised on sustainable farms is the same as that of livestock raised in CAFOs: to be finished and killed for meat. But while they're alive, animals on sustainable, pasture-based farms are given the chance to live more natural lives.

Free-range eggs come from hens that are allowed to roam. The phrase "free-range eggs" sounds goofy, as if the eggs themselves have been ranging freely, exuberantly rolling around the pasture. Of course, it's the hens that are allowed to range free, pecking the ground, eating grasshoppers and worms and dead baby rabbits that the cats leave lying around. Our free-range chickens aren't that easy to keep alive, basically because everything out there wants to eat them: weasels, coyotes, dogs, hawks, eagles, cats. Free-range hens come into the barn at night to get up on their roosts, and we shut the door against predators.

Free-range hens don't always follow the rules. They are supposed to lay their eggs in nest boxes. This way every day we can gather eggs from the boxes. Of course, if a hen is on the nest, she won't appreciate my groping around underneath her. In fact, as I reach under, she'll give a low growl-cackle in her throat, half threatening, half indignant. It's warm and soft and plump under the hen, and though I'm tempted to leave my hand there awhile to warm up, I don't, basically because the hen is pecking an impressive ring of blood around my wrist.

Taped to the door of our chicken room is a blown-up Dan Piraro cartoon that shows a dour farmer in bib overalls and straw hat holding a basket of eggs, chatting with his hen. "Kristine, I had originally intended to kill and eat you. But since we've become so close, I've decided to just steal your children every day and have them for breakfast instead."

Poor Kristine. But when you take an egg away, she'll lay another in a day or two. And she wants to sit on anything as long as it's egg-shaped. Put a plastic Easter egg in the nest box, and she'll sit on it. Put a wooden egg in the nest box, and she'll sit on it. Sometimes when I swipe an egg from under a hen, I feel bad, so I'll replace it with a wooden egg from another nest, and she'll happily reach for it with her beak, rolling it underneath her. Give a hen a duck egg, a goose egg, an ostrich egg, and if she can fit it underneath her, it's hers.

We keep the hens locked up for the morning, hoping to force them to deposit their eggs in the nest boxes. But at noon, when I let them out, a few of them head for their secret hiding places, which might be in a box, under a bench, maybe behind a bin or a stack of pallets. Hens are so resourceful at hiding their eggs that we may not find them until the summer day one of us walks through the tall grass behind the barn and steps right into a stash of thirty eggs.

Some hens are unable to keep quiet about the good news. Once she's laid her egg in this secret place, she stands up, flaps her wings, and cackles happily. It's as if a pirate buried his treasure, then stood directly over it, jumping up and down and telling the other pirates he's buried a great treasure. This may be why chickens have a reputation for not being the brightest lightbulbs in the barn.

The eggs we gather from these chickens are as fresh as you can get. How fresh are store eggs? Eggs sold to consumers must be packaged within twenty-one days of being laid, then will likely have another thirty days before they expire, although this is just for eggs from USDA-inspected plants. According to the American Egg Board, cartons from USDA-inspected plants must display a Julian date—the date the eggs were packed. Unfortunately, the Julian date is a confusing string of numbers that are unrecognizable as a date, at least to me.

While a fifty-one-day-old egg is still perfectly edible, by then the yolks are pale yellow and the whites are runny. As an egg ages, water from the outer edges of the egg migrates to the yolk, thereby weakening the yolk, which is why you can break the yolk from an old egg just by staring at it. Eat a fresh egg and you'll be alarmed at how the yolk sits up, plump and high, and screams, "I am orange, *really* orange!" Even better, studies have shown that pasture chickens lay eggs that have 10 percent less total fat, 40 percent more vitamin A, 400 percent more omega-3s, and 34 percent less cholesterol than factory eggs.[4] According to *Mother Earth News,* expert bakers swear by pasture-raised eggs, some saying that the firm, fresh eggs give their cakes 30 percent more lift.

Decoding the labels on egg cartons is a challenge, since I haven't actually purchased eggs this way in twelve years, but a number of sources seem to agree that labels break down as below:

**Certified Organic:** These eggs have been certified by a program approved by the U.S. Department of Agriculture to have been laid by hens fed only organic feed, not given antibiotics, nor kept in cages. Debeaking is allowed. Access to the outdoors is apparently still a topic of hot debate.

**Certified Humane:** These eggs are from chickens certified by Humane Farm Animal Care to be uncaged, with access to perches, nest boxes, and dust for bathing. Outdoor access isn't required, and debeaking is allowed.

**Cage free, Free range, or Free-roaming:** Mindy Pennybacker, editor of *The Green Guide* (http://thegreenguide.com) warns that these are among the least reliable labels, since they are poorly defined and not verified by any certification organization. Cage-free usually means the hens are not in cages, but are in large open buildings and able to walk around and stretch their legs a bit, although there could be ten thousand chickens in a building. Some may have been "allowed access to the outside," but this doesn't necessarily mean they take advantage of it. If a chicken has been raised most of its life inside, and you suddenly open a door to the outside, it may not go through it. Inside is safe and known; outside is scary and unknown.

**Omega-3:** This has more to do with the egg's content than how the hen was cared for. All eggs contain some omega-3 fatty acids. You can crank up the omega-3 in an egg by feeding the hens fish oil, flaxseed, or by letting them forage out on pasture.[5]

••• ••• •••

Chickens raised outside, whether they are layers or broilers, face a constant threat from predators. You could let 500 chickens out into the pasture, but unless they have a safe place for sleeping at night, you'll have only 490 the next morning. Do the math, and you'll be out of business very quickly as every fox, coyote, hawk, owl, or dog in the neighborhood stops by with all its friends for a late evening snack.

Some farmers protect their broiler chickens by raising them in floorless pens that are moved every day. The chickens never get out of the pens, but they have fresh grass between their chicken toes, fresh grass to eat, and fresh grass to poop on.

Other farmers devise small sheds, letting the chickens roam around during the day (a chicken won't range all that far away from its food source, water, and safe sleeping spot), and then at dusk, after the chickens have returned to the shed, the farmer shuts the door. It's best if this enclosure can be moved every now and then, since the chickens will make a mess of the area around the little building.

A sustainable farmer knows she's going to lose some chickens to predators; you just want to keep the losses as low as possible. We had what we suspected was a mink that visited our broiler pens every night, managing to reach under the cage's bottom edge, snag a chicken, and pull the chicken's head under the cage. Day after day we'd find headless chickens just inside the pen. It was most disturbing. This is probably why it's hard to find meat chickens that are free-ranging. The farmer needs to have something left to sell at the end of the day.

When we started raising laying hens, I had been stunned to learn that chickens are omnivores. If it's moving, a chicken will peck at it. If it's not moving, a chicken will peck at it. They love to chase down grasshoppers or crickets. They'll fight over a worm, tugging on each end until, well, there are suddenly two worms. Chickens eat grain, but they also eat meat—any meat. Put a dead mouse in the chicken house, and there won't be much left in an hour. We often joke as one of us heads out the door. "I'm going into the chicken house. If I'm not back in fifteen minutes, come looking for me." It's best not to lose consciousness and fall to the floor in the chicken house.

What does it mean to be a chicken? I watch ours and marvel at their ability to seek out and find bugs. They eat seeds. They eat grass. They eat my flowers. They clean up the grain a goat has spilled. They like to find a patch of softer soil and dig a small depression. Here they burrow down and flap their wings, getting dust under their feathers to dry out any external parasites nibbling on them. They sit in the sun and fall asleep. They stretch out, one leg extended, one wing extended, and you can just tell it feels good.

••• ••• •••

Like humans and chickens, hogs are also omnivorous, which means a steady diet of nothing but grass won't work for them. So don't look too hard for entirely grass-fed pork or grass-finished pork. But sustainable farms with pasture-based systems do let hogs be hogs. Pigs wallow in the mud not because they're dirty creatures but because pigs don't have sweat glands, so mud helps keep pigs cool and protects their skin from sunburn and bug bites. Pigs also like to go swimming. I love Michael Sowa's painting of a lovely lake scene with a dock, trees, and blue sky. In the center of this idyllic scene, leaping off the dock with great exuberance, is a pig.

Pigs are curious and use their big snouts to explore. Not only does the pig use its great sense of smell to do this, but the snout has the sensitivity of a human hand. Pigs are highly social animals, living naturally in groups of three to five adult sows and their young. They are intelligent and playful. Shannon Hayes writes: "They're a joy to watch as they run around, chase each other, splash in their wallows, squeal as the farmer prepares their food, chase toys. . . . Throw them a ball and they will be amused for hours."[6] Pigs are naturally clean animals, preferring not to excrete near their living and eating areas, and only become overweight when overfed by their human caretakers.

About twenty-four hours before giving birth, a sow will find a spot, make a hole in the ground, and build a nest using whatever she can find. The sow's instinct to nest is incredibly powerful. Our friend Dale, who'd been raised on a hog farm, tells the story of one sow that ripped off a wooden gate and broke it apart for her base. Then she dragged over a pile of corncobs from the cattle's feed trough. She broke into another part of the barn and dragged an entire bale of straw back to her nest, breaking it apart and fluffing it up into a comfy nest. She climbed on board and gave birth to a litter of piglets.

Unfortunately, this was in the winter, and she'd built this nest outside in the middle of the cattle pen, with no protection from the elements. Dale and his family had quite a time getting this protective mama and her babies into a more sheltered spot, and I think it involved calming the angry sow down with—wait for it—a bottle of beer. Christopher Hogwood was not alone in his love of the hops.

Many sustainable farmers raise hogs out on pasture using the system Tom Frantzen had observed in Sweden, the open-ended hoop houses with lots of straw for bedding, and manure in the bedding composts providing a source of warmth for the animals. The sows have material for making nests when they're ready. The animals don't come down with respiratory problems, because the fresh air moves so easily through the hoop houses. The animals have plenty of room and an environment that stimulates that curious snout. A hog pasture field won't look as lovely and uniform as my sheep pasture, but more like a minefield from all the rooting.

•••  •••  •••

The life of beef cattle on a sustainable farm is relatively simple: graze, graze, graze. They may live in a feedlot in the winter, or the farmer may leave them out on pasture and bring the hay to them. I've seen photos of farmers who take those seven-hundred-to-thirteen-hundred-pound big round bales and unroll them like you'd unroll ribbon, and then the cattle eat the hay directly off the snow. It will take longer to raise a beef steer up to market weight on a grass-based diet, because the farmer isn't feeding it buckets of grain every day or pumping it full of hormones or antibiotics.

Our steer lives a good life. He doesn't have the wooly protection the sheep do, so he has fulltime access to the barn in the winter. Most farmers, both sustainable and conventional, do this, because an animal that is desperately cold will not eat as well nor gain weight as well as an animal that's more comfortable.

Sustainable dairies present interesting challenges. By its very nature, a dairy must keep animals closer together. It can't be moving its herd from pasture to pasture as we do our sheep, since those cows must be milked twice a day, and on large farms you'd end up spending your whole day moving them back and forth. But sustainable dairies find a way, because they recognize that grazing their animals is important both to animal health and to the quality of their products. They will likely market their products as grass-fed, or organic, or free from rBST.

We toured an organic dairy where after grazing a pasture the cows used an underpass below the road to return to the milking barn. Those cows were big, glossy, calm, and I wanted to take them home with us.

•••   •••   •••

Sustainable farming is about relationships: a farmer's relationship with animals; a farmer's relationships with the people buying the meat, eggs, or dairy products; and a farmer's relationship with the environment. I love how Roger Scruton describes the life of a livestock farmer:

> Livestock farming is not merely an industry—it is a relation, in which man and animal are bound together to their mutual profit, and in which a human duty of care is nourished by an animal's mute recognition of dependency. There is something consoling and heart warming in the proximity of contented herbivores, in the rituals of feeding them, catching them, and coaxing them from field to field. This partly explains why people will continue in this time-consuming, exhausting and ill-paid occupation, resisting the attempts by bureaucrats and agribusiness to drive them to extinction.[7]

Whether you call them sustainable farms, organic farms, or small family farms, most small farmers—sustainable and conventional alike—care deeply for their animals. They want to give their animals a life that's as good as possible. Maybe there's some hope for Old MacDonald's farm after all.

# Go Organic . . .
# or Not

••• ••• •••••• ••• •••

EPICUREANS BELIEVED IN the austere life and simple food, yet centuries later the word *epicurean* has been twisted around to mean "devoted to the pursuit of sensual pleasure, especially to the enjoyment of good food." I think of fancy food, gourmet food. While the word *organic* hasn't been entirely stood on its head like *epicurean,* it's certainly been tipped a bit.

Everyone seems to agree on the basic definition of organic: food grown without the assistance of man-made chemicals. Organic means natural, good, and wholesome. Thousands of produce farmers work very hard to raise fruits and vegetables organically, and they deserve a great deal of credit for educating consumers about the health and environmental benefits of going organic. They are why organic is now the fastest-growing segment of the food industry. Since 1990 the growth in organic food sales has exceeded 20 percent a year, compared to 1 percent in the overall food industry. Sales in 2005 were $14 billion. The Organic Trade Association predicts the market will grow 11 percent per year through 2010.[8] Not surprisingly, these sorts of numbers attract big business.

As organic gets really big, it faces the same questions every growing industry faces: what now? Here's what the Organic Trade Association had to say:

> As food companies scramble to find enough organically grown in-gredients, they are inevitably forsaking the pastoral ethos that has defined the organic lifestyle. For some companies, it means keep-ing thousands of organic cows on industrial-scale feedlots. For others, the scarcity of organic ingredients means looking as far afield as China, Sierra Leone, and Brazil—places where standards may be hard to enforce, workers' wages and living conditions are a worry, and, say critics, increased farmland sometimes comes at a cost to the environment.[9]

*Organic* no longer describes a philosophy or an approach to food. It is a legal term describing food that has been certified by the USDA as organic, meaning "a production system that is managed to respond to site-specific conditions by integrating cultural, bio-logical, and mechanical practices that foster cycling of resources, promote ecological balance and conserve biodiversity." Say what?

For meat to be certified by the USDA as organic, these condi-tions must be met:

- Animals for slaughter must be raised under organic management from the last third of gestation, or no later than the second day of life for poultry.
- Livestock feed must be 100 percent organic.
- No hormones or antibiotics are allowed, although vac-cines are allowed. Any animal treated with a prohib-ited medication may not be sold as organic.

- Farmers must treat sick animals even if it means the animal will lose its organic status.
- The animals must have access to the outdoors; ruminants must have access to pasture.

You've probably noticed that these standards are the same as those that most sustainable farmers follow, the main exception being the 100 percent organic feed. And while the guidelines require that animals have "access to pasture," they don't say how much or for how long. As a result, animals can be kept on huge feedlots yet become dairy and meat products that can be labeled organic.

Author Joan Dye Gussow wrote in *Organic Gardening*: "This isn't what we meant. . . . When we said organic, we meant local. We meant healthful. We meant being true to the ecologies of regions. We meant mutually respectful growers and eaters. We meant social justice and community."[10]

When people hear how we farm, their first question is almost more of a statement: "You're an organic farm, then." Well, no. We can't call ourselves organic unless we jump through the USDA's paper hoops and comply with all the regulations.

Some of us don't like jumping through hoops. Some of us are unable to find a source for 100 percent organic feed for our livestock. Melissa and I tried and tried and finally gave up, running into too many delivery and cost obstacles.

As a result, there are thousands of small farms that raise animals according to the old-fashioned organic *principles* yet cannot legally call themselves organic. It's great that people have finally caught on to the idea of organic food, and I want to take nothing away from those farmers who have successfully gone organic, but it's a bit frustrating that many consumers now believe that only food labeled organic is any good. Perhaps we need to separate the idea of an organic system from the idea of legally organic food.

Farmers, and the U.S. government, take this new definition of organic very seriously, as they should, since there's no point in having a standard if the consumer can't trust that the farm actually meets those standards without tramping out to the farm himself. If I sell less than five thousand dollars' worth of meat a year, and follow the standards, I may legally call my lamb organic. But if I sell more than five thousand dollars per year, it's the certification process for me. The consequences of skipping that whole paperwork scene? As the Sustainable Agriculture Network (SAN) explains, "A civil penalty of up to $10,000 can be levied on any person who knowingly sells or labels as organic a product that is not produced and handled in accordance with the National Organic Program regulations."[11]

In the fall of 2007 the USDA announced actions taken against Aurora Organic Dairy in Boulder, Colorado, the country's largest organic factory dairy, as a result of complaints filed that the dairy has been flooding the market with "bogus organic milk," driving down the prices paid to ethical organic farmers. The animals have been confined in feedlots (up to five thousand cows in one of the company's facilities) with no access to pasture, and the company has been purchasing nonorganic feed and representing its milk as organic when it didn't legally qualify.[12]

Bill Niman of Niman Ranch, one of the most impressive success stories of marketing sustainably raised meat from a network of small farms, chooses not to "go organic" because he believes that there isn't enough organic grain to feed both humans and livestock, and that the priority should be feeding humans, not animals, with the organic grain. Also, organic grain raises the price of organic meat, which might put his meat out of reach of too many consumers.[13] As author Nina Planck has said, "I seldom look for the organic label on beef and butter. 'Grass fed' means a lot more. . . . These foods—and others raised with ecological and humane methods—are superior to industrial organic foods. The Agriculture Department may never tell you that, but smart farmers will."[14]

The legal labeling of organic meat is a good thing because it helps build trust between you and the farmer. But keep in mind that not all sustainable farmers choose to go organic. And not all organic farms are small farms. I hate to start beating a drum others have pounded so thoroughly before me, but E. F. Schumacher might have been right when he wrote that "small is beautiful"— small organic farms, small sustainable farms, even small conventional farms.

# To Certify or
# Not to Certify

••• ••• •••••• ••• •••

WHILE ORGANIC IS the most well known certification, humane certifications are being offered, too. These certifications may help customers judge a food's origins when they can't visit the farm, but once again it's unwise for consumers to believe that *only* certified humane farms are good farms, or that *only* certified organic farms are good farms. There are many reasons why small farmers don't seek humane certification.

For example, I came across an exciting new certification program called "Animal Welfare Approved Standards for Sheep."[15] Developed by the Animal Welfare Institute (AWI), I thought this might be a good thing for us to consider and apply for, adding weight to our assertions that we raise our animals humanely.

I flew to the AWI Web site, my fingers atremble, and began reading.

"The natural environment and artificial shelter for animals must allow the animals to behave naturally, performing behaviors essential to each animal's psychological and physical health and well-being. The system must be fitted to the animal, rather than the animal fitted to the system." Yes, I can see the AWI is riding the same train I am. Work *with* nature rather than against her.

"Shepherds must ensure that the sheep, including lambs from two weeks of age, have continuous access to pastures of good grazing and nutrient quality unless freezing or snow cover prevent grazing." Again, yes. Get the animals out of the barn and onto pasture. Let them run around and be animals. Let them harvest their own food.

"Lambing shall take place out on pasture." I swell with pride. The AWI surely must have used our farm as a guide.

The guidelines kept getting better, suggesting lambs not be weaned until they are five months old—about when we wean them. By then the ewes have gotten fed up with lambs bashing their udders and have mostly weaned the lambs themselves. Sheep should always have fresh water, a given on our farm. Melissa has a water-level detector built into her brain, so whenever the water level falls an inch, a beeper sounds in her head and she rushes out to top off the water buckets.

But the more I read, the more statements I found that began to disturb me. "Whether or not guard or herd dogs will be permitted is under AWI review due to the fact that sheep can demonstrate anti-predator responses to dogs." Good lord! That's the whole point of using a herding dog—to make the sheep uncomfortable so they will run from the dog into the correct pen or pasture. Being herded by a dog is part of a sheep's life. As for guard dogs, they live with the flock and frighten off coyotes or other predators. Guard dogs aren't scary to the sheep because they've been living with the flock since they were puppies. The dog-question statement is no longer on the Web site, so hopefully they've let go of the idea that sheep dogs should be banned from sheep farms.

"All animals must be able to lie down comfortably during transport." What's comfortably? Our lambs have a forty-minute drive, and we pack them into the trailer because they are safer this way. With too much room, animals can be tossed about or knocked over as the trailer turns corners or stops suddenly.

I reached the shelter criteria. "Animals must have continuous, unobstructed access to shelter, either natural or artificial. . . . The shelter shall protect sheep from weather extremes that could endanger their health and well-being."

Continuous access to shelter is nearly impossible on a pasture-based farm. When the shepherd moves the sheep to fresh grass every day, she is moving the sheep farther and farther from the barn. Is she being cruel? No, because here's the thing: sheep carry their shelter with them. If you were covered in five inches of wool, you'd understand. Sheep can lie out in the middle of a snowstorm chewing their cuds. The next morning oval prints mark where their body heat melted the snow all the way down to bare ground. When it's raining, they turn their butts to the rain and just wait for it to stop, or they lie down and catch a bit of shut-eye.

In the north there are two circumstances when shelter is necessary. We shear our sheep in March, and it's still cold. So they have twenty-four-hour access to the barn for a few weeks until the weather warms up. The other time the sheep need shelter is on a ninety-five-degree day in the middle of July. For that, we provide an old hay wagon, our pickup truck, and other shelters, or we move the sheep into pastures with trees so that they'll be in shade.

But the AWI standards insist the sheep have access to shelter all the time. Unless a farmer is independently wealthy and can afford to build shelters all over his farm, how could this ever happen? We have more than fifteen different sections to our pasture—do we build a barn in each one? I don't think so.

A portable shelter, you suggest. Big enough for one hundred sheep? How do you move it? What about the fact that our pastures are hilly? Suddenly we're talking about spending hours every

day moving shelters for the sheep. If the shelters were truly necessary, we'd figure something out. But they just aren't necessary.

AWI standards also say, "Tail docking is prohibited. Shepherds
must find other ways to prevent blowflies from laying eggs that
will develop into maggots, under the tail." Unlike animals in a
barn, animals on pasture cannot be easily caught, examined, and
treated every day. The only part of a sheep's tail we are likely to
see is the tip as she's running away from us. (But now the sheep is
exhibiting anti-predator behavior, because I scared it, so the cynic
in me wonders if perhaps shepherds themselves should be banned
from sheep farms.)

To dock a tail, some farmers cut it off. Others slide a tight rubber band onto the tail, cutting off blood circulation to the tail so
that it eventually atrophies and falls off. Shepherds who raise
sheep for the show ring take off so much of the tail that the rectal
muscles are adversely affected, leading to rectal prolapses. But
those of us raising animals for meat on pasture leave enough of
the tail to avoid that problem.

Why dock tails? Because in this area warm, moist weather
brings out the flies, and they look for places that are rich in nutrients in which to lay their eggs. If a sheep has diarrhea, the manure tends to cling to the wool around the tail, and the flies head
straight for her. And who is to say which is more stressful—the
numbness from the rubber band, or the terrible itching that
lambs experience when maggots begin consuming their flesh?

I keep finding books written by interviewing authors who
pounce on farmers with this question: "And you do this proce-
dure without anesthesia?" The farmers never have a good answer,
because the question doesn't make any sense to them. We do occasionally cause an animal pain or stress, but the expense and
time of administering some sort of anesthesia isn't practical.

As a farmer I do not want to cause my animals any unnecessary
pain or suffering, but I cannot guarantee a totally pain-free life.

There must be some balance between treating the animal like a treasured pet, complete with pink collar and cute name, and treating that animal like nothing more than a plastic widget. I hope that, as a farmer, I have a realistic relationship with my livestock.

Our animals will experience mild pain now and then, since we give them shots. We put tags through their ears. We dock the tails of all our lambs. Do those little lambs lie around and moan in pain for days? Nope, they run off and thirty minutes later are jumping up and down, running around Mama, leaping on her sleeping back, and basically having a great time. I'm basing my opinions not on scientific studies of whether an animal feels pain, or on how much, but on observation. The pain fades.

Scientist and author Temple Grandin believes animals have higher tolerances for pain, but lower tolerances for fear, than humans do. "Animals in terrible pain can still function; they can function so well they can act as if nothing in the world is wrong. An animal in a state of panic can't function at all."[16] I don't want my animals to be in either a state of panic or in terrible pain, and we do our absolute best to make sure neither happens.

There may be other things farmers do to their animals that you wish they wouldn't do. Sometimes an animal must be penned up separately. It might be sick, and the farmer doesn't want it to infect the entire flock or herd while it recovers. When we isolate an animal, we do our best to make sure it can at least see another animal so it won't be frightened.

We trim our sheep's hooves. This requires that we restrain them in a metal cage and tip them back onto their butts so that we can deal with their feet. Do they enjoy this little carnival ride? No, but it's either that or have them walk painfully on hooves curled up like ski tips.

Certification will often be the only way a consumer has to judge the products she faces on the grocery shelf, but the programs aren't perfect. Don't exclude perfectly fine meat raised by farmers who aren't certified. As I'll discuss later, visit the farms or meet the farmers, and verify they are raising their animals in a way you can support.

I don't need my meat to come from animals that lived an entire life without pain or fear, since I now know that's almost impossible to deliver. What's more important to me is that domestic livestock be raised as living, breathing creatures with emotions and needs, not as inputs in a widget factory. On that, the AWI and I agree.

# An Animal Is
# What It Eats

... ... ...... ... ...

THE FEED A farmer puts in her animal's mouth ends up going one of two places: some comes out the other end, and some becomes part of the animal's body, including the muscle, or flesh. And since we eat that flesh, it makes sense that what I feed my animals affects how that animal tastes. I don't mean to complicate things, but just choosing a farm type for your meat isn't the end of it, since each type of farm can finish its animals any number of ways. A more conscious carnivore needs to pay attention to the feeding options, how that feed affects the animal's health, and how that feed affects the taste.

Imagine a continuum with all grain on one end, and all grass on the other. Factory farms feed their animals nearly all grain. Some sustainable farmers feed their animals only grass. The rest of us—conventional, sustainable, and organic—can fall anywhere along that continuum. Also, *grass* is a catchall term for anything green. Agricultural folks call these forages, but the word has never stuck in my brain. Grass can be alfalfa, clover, bird's-foot trefoil, and dozens of different types of grass.

First, a brief commercial for the rumen, part of the amazing system that takes the green plants we can't eat and turns them into animal flesh, which we can. Ruminants are animals that have a stomach with four compartments, and that regurgitate their food to have another go at chewing it up. The definition of ruminate is to "chew again what has been chewed slightly and swallowed." Nummy. Humans, thank heavens, have only one stomach. Pigs and chickens are not ruminants, so they can't survive on grass alone.

The four compartments, or stomachs, of ruminant animals are the rumen, reticulum, omasum, and abomasum. The grazing sheep chews the food a bit, then swallows it, where it sits in the rumen, getting all soft, thanks to saliva and the beginnings of digestion, then it heads for the reticulum. When a sheep feels full, it's time to find a spot in the sun, lie down, and regurgitate the half-chewed grass and chew it again. This is what an animal is doing when she's chewing her cud. After the cud's all nicely chewed up, the animal swallows and the food zips through the rumen and reticulum into the omasum for more processing. Finally it hits the true stomach—the abomasum—where acids and digestive enzymes do their thing and release the nutrients from the chewed food.

Cows spend six hours a day eating and about eight hours a day chewing their cud, and it impresses me that a ruminant's jaw can withstand that sort of constant activity without orthodontic help.

How does this digestive system get off balance? An animal's rumen contains microbes with the important job of breaking down the food so that the animal can absorb, process, or eliminate what needs to be absorbed, processed, or eliminated. But with the wrong feed, this process falters.

In factory feedlots the goal is to feed as many calories as possible to get the animal up to market weight as quickly, and as cheaply, as possible. As Michael Pollan brought to our attention in *The Omnivore's Dilemma*, when it comes to calories, corn is king. Unfortunately, when fed a heavy corn diet, most cattle today get sick.

The heavy corn diet creates such acid in their bodies that their livers blow out. A steady diet of antibiotics is the only way feedlot owners can keep the cattle alive long enough to get them up to market weight. One vet told Pollan, "Hell, if you gave them [the cattle] lots of grass and space, I wouldn't have a job."[17]

A more natural diet for ruminants is all grass, or grass with a small amount of grain. You'll see farmers and stores and markets selling grass-fed and grass-finished foods. Because the government hasn't yet gotten around to regulating us graziers, there aren't set legal definitions for these terms. I've used *grass-fed* to mean the animal ate grass at some point in its life, and *grass-finished* to mean that in the last few months of an animal's life it ate *only* grass. Unfortunately, I've come across pasture-focused Web sites that switch these two definitions around, so the best way to be sure is to ask the farmer directly.

The diet for pasture-raised beef and sheep will vary from farm to farm, and there isn't any one right way to do this, but the diet for our steer will be considerably different than in a factory feedlot. Instead of 95 percent grain, the diet will probably be less than 40 percent grain, and the roughage—in the form of grass or hay—will help the rumen work correctly. Many sustainable farmers feed grain to their animals. Grain, in itself, isn't bad—it's the scale that's important. Too much grain, and you have an unhealthy animal. Too much grain, and you have meat laced with fat. Too much grain, and the farmer uses lots of fossil fuel to raise and transport that grain instead of relying on the grass growing under the animal's hooves.

In the three months before slaughter, we feed each of our lambs about one pound of corn a day, which is a small percentage of their total diet, but for some pasture purists, any grain is wrong. We do it because it yields a meat product we enjoy, it makes the animals happy, and it gives them some extra energy during the winter. An animal less stressed by cold will grow faster.

The beef industry has successfully developed a grain-fed product that's fairly consistent across the country, so we're all used to the same taste. A hamburger in Atlanta won't taste that different from one in Seattle. But grass-fed meat tastes different than grain-fed meat, which is why people have widely varying reactions to meat from animals raised on grass. The first time I bit into a grass-fed steak, I was stunned. It didn't taste like anything I was used to. I didn't like it, because I'd expected it to taste exactly like the corn-fed beef I've eaten all my life.

I know now I'd been going about it all wrong. A chef giving a cooking demonstration at a recent Grazefest (a fun event where you can tour a farm, eat pasture-raised food, and come face-to-face with a cow) explained that the best way to approach eating grass-fed meat is to think of it as an entirely different animal so you'll be more open to a different taste. Grass-fed meat tastes wonderful, as long as you don't expect it to taste just like grain-finished. That's the same approach adventurous carnivores use when they try bison or elk or venison, or (dare I say it?) lamb. All of these meats taste different than grain-finished beef.

We've been feeding our steer ten pounds of whole corn a day, and he's been grazing on the green stuff. We don't know if the meat will taste more like corn-fed or more like grass-fed; we're expecting it to be somewhere in between. Learning from our experiences takes time.

A compassionate carnivore recognizes the link between what an animal eats and how it tastes, and accepts that you have the right to find some balance between these factors. If you try grass-finished meat and love it, no problem. But if you don't love it, don't give up and think that your only choice is to return to factory meat. Try it again. If it's still not what you want, there are many farmers, and animals, who fall somewhere between these two extremes. You just might need to do a little hoof work (sorry, I couldn't resist!) to find them.

# To Your
# Health

••• ••• •••••• ••• •••

FOR SOME OF you, health might be a factor or motivator when it comes to buying meat. For me, health really isn't as important as the other issues, since I've lived through so many food scares and health claims that I don't pay much attention to them anymore. But studies do show that grass-fed meat has less overall fat. A 2002 study in the *European Journal of Clinical Nutrition* found that meat from grass-fed animals not only contained less fat, but also that the fat was healthier. Grass-fed meat contains up to four times as much beta-carotene as factory meat, which helps maintain healthy vision and lowers the risk of breast cancer. The increased carotene results in colored fat, from "a creamy hue to almost yellow," reports Jo Robinson in *Pasture Perfect.*[18] In countries where animals are still raised predominately on grass, white fat is considered freakish. As a chef in Argentina observed, "Looking at the fat of a USDA Choice steak is like looking at the face of a dead man."[19]

Whoa.

Grass-fed meat has more omega-3 fatty acids, which help lower cholesterol. Animals raised in factories accumulate omega-6 fatty acids, the "bad" fats, which have been linked to cancer, diabetes, obesity, and immune disorders.[20] Grass-fed meat contains from three to six times more vitamin E than factory meat.[21]

Grass-fed meat contains more conjugated linoleic acid (CLA), a fat that helps fight cancer and cardiovascular disease. Meat from animals raised on grass contains two to five times the amount of CLA as meat from grain-fed animals.

Those who eat grass-fed meat can relax a bit about always choosing chicken over beef, since according to the *Journal of Animal Science,* grass-fed beef has the same amount of fat as a chicken breast but more omega-3s.[22] So a grass-fed steak might be healthier than factory-raised chicken.

As for factory meat, what the owners put into the animals ends up, not surprisingly, in the meat. Tufts University researchers have shown that human exposure to the endocrine-disrupting hormones given to cattle can increase the risk of breast and ovarian cancer in women and testicular cancer in men, as well as reduce sperm quality and count.[23] Because of the potential side effects of hormones, including intestinal cancers and premature puberty, the European Union banned them in 1988. We in the United States still use them.[24]

Arsenic is fed to 70 percent of the chickens in the United States, mixed in with antibiotics and feed to promote growth and prevent illness.[25] In 2006 the Institute for Agriculture and Trade Policy tested chicken meat in supermarkets and restaurants and found that 75 percent of the chicken contained detectable levels of arsenic.[26] The levels of arsenic in chicken meat wouldn't normally be a problem, but remember we're eating more chicken than ever before, so we're ingesting more arsenic. Tyson Foods, the nation's largest chicken producer, stopped feeding arsenic to its chickens in 2004, but many other processors still use it.[27]

While hormones and arsenic are *inside* the factory meat, an even greater threat is what's on the outside of the meat. In July 2002 the USDA announced the recall of 19 million pounds of ground beef that may have been contaminated with E. coli. Twenty-seven people in seven states fell ill. The largest recall ever was in 1997, when 25 million pounds were recalled.[28] The National Centers for Disease Control estimates that every year four thousand Americans die and five million get sick from eating contaminated meat.[29]

Where are these contaminants coming from? When fed almost nothing but grain, the pH in a cow's rumen drops. Scientists believe a new strain of E. coli discovered in 1993 developed in this highly acidic environment. While our own stomach acids successfully killed off the common E. coli years ago, this new strain is proving much more resistant, because our stomachs aren't acidic enough to kill it.

E. coli makes its way from the rumen into the animal's manure and onto its hide. Sloppy slaughterhouse practices allow manure from the animal's hide to touch the meat, and if not cleaned off, E. coli may remain on the outside of the muscle.

If we cook our steaks and roasts properly, the E. coli is destroyed. But when it comes to ground beef, the act of grinding mixes up the E. coli with all the meat, and it becomes part of the interior of a hamburger. If that burger isn't cooked to a high enough temperature, the E. coli will survive and possibly end up in someone's stomach, where stomach acids are no match for this super strain.

The more grain an animal eats, the greater potential for E. coli to take up residence in its body. Eating grass keeps an animal's rumen in better balance, which is good for the animal, and good for your health.

••• ••• •••

Melissa and I used to belong to a grazing group (once again, farmers who graze animals, not who themselves graze!). Once a month we'd visit a member's farm and tour the pasture. The plant enthusiasts, which included Melissa, would end up staring down at a patch of grass for what felt like hours, totally absorbed in discussing the plants growing there. After an hour of this, a few of us non-grass fanatics would roll our eyes and head back to the house for food. I am, after all, my father's daughter and don't get much of an adrenaline rush from discussing the growth patterns of brome grass versus timothy.

As a carnivore who is concerned about the environment and your health, you don't need to know if that patch of ground contains red clover or alsike clover, or if the bird's-foot trefoil is re-seeding itself, or if the animals find the fescue unpalatable this year. You just need to know that when it comes to feeding livestock, grass is as green as it gets.

Part Five

# Choosing How
# Animals Die

When you have to make a choice and don't make it,
that is in itself a choice.

—WILLIAM JAMES

There's one more piece to the puzzle of deciding which meat to consume, and this is the piece most of us tenderhearted animal lovers want to avoid. We've looked away for most of our lives, but if we're to become more compassionate meat eaters, willing to pay attention and take responsibility for our actions, we need to face how an animal dies.

I have never seen one of my animals butchered. When I began this book, I thought that perhaps I needed to take this step to somehow prove to myself I was a "real" farmer, a stalwart soul, able to face unflinchingly every step of the process. Besides, if urban meat eaters were willing to step outside their comfort zones by acknowledging that they were eating animals, and by getting to know those animals better and taking some responsibility for the quality of the animals' lives, surely I could watch an animal being butchered, a simple act that humans have witnessed for thousands and thousands of years without undue psychological damage.

Or maybe not.

So far, I haven't, and that's okay. But if I choose not to kill my own meat, and choose not to witness someone else doing it, then what's left? To educate myself about the process, to acknowledge that an animal is being killed to feed me, and to use my meat dollars to support the way I'd rather have animals butchered on my behalf.

When it comes to livestock and meat, to *butcher* means "to slaughter, skin, remove the entrails, and cut up the carcass for meat." The other dictionary definitions, like "to kill in a barbarous manner" or "to botch something," don't really apply, or so I thought. But when I began looking into how animals raised in factories are killed in gigantic slaughterhouses using inhumane production lines, it hit me. All three definitions do indeed apply.

# Where There's Livestock, There's Dead Stock

••• ••• •••••• ••• •••

I'VE NEVER SEEN an animal butchered, but I have seen plenty of dead animals and have held dying animals in my arms. Death is such a part of farming that weary farmers have a saying: where there's livestock, there's gonna be dead stock.

There are a discouragingly large number of ways animals can die. *Sheep Industry News* now and then runs a table of sheep death loss by cause. Predators are number one, followed by old age, but other causes include digestive problems (bloat, scours, parasites, enterotoxemia), respiratory problems, metabolic problems (milk fever, pregnancy toxemia), weather-related events (drowning, lightning), theft, poisoning (nitrate poisoning, noxious feeds, noxious weeds), and lambing problems.[1] Even in the best of environments, and under the best of care, it's a challenge to keep animals alive.

If an animal becomes ill and the farmer doesn't notice, the animal might die from a treatable disease. An animal can contract a fatal disease and die a long, slow death, or die a quick one if the farmer knows how to use a gun, wield a knife, or has the money to bring the vet out with the required needle and deadly syringe. Unfortunately, once an animal looks sick, many farmers ship it off to the livestock market to be purchased and dealt with by someone else.

Not all animals survive their own births. We've had stillborn lambs. We've had lambs die from lack of oxygen when something goes wrong during the birth. A newborn lamb is amazingly hearty, up on its feet and nursing quickly, some within thirty minutes. They get command of their wobbly legs and within a few hours can hop a bit or run a short way. Despite their strength, however, now and then a lamb will get pneumonia, strong and robust one day and dead the next. Sheep have a clever protection against predators—they hide their illnesses, since a predator scanning a flock will most likely pick out animals that look weak and sick. This inborn protection works, but it also means farmers often don't know an animal is sick. We've learned to watch the sheep's ears. They should be pointing straight out from the sides of the head. If they're down, the animal's really sick. Melissa tries valiantly to save every sick animal, but we've come to accept that at least with sheep, by the time they reveal they are ill, it's often too late.

Weather can kill. Our ram Monte appeared perfectly healthy, but something must have been wrong inside him, so even though he had plenty of water, grass, and shade, a July heat wave proved deadly. Melissa found the 250-pound ram dead in the shade.

Every winter Minnesota usually has a nasty streak of dangerously cold weather, twenty degrees below zero, with a minus-forty windchill. Even though our sheep are protected by five inches of wool, can get out of the wind, and have plenty of food and water, the cold can stress an animal. One of our original ewes, eleven years old and slowing down a bit, died in the barn during a recent cold snap. Death is a perfectly natural part of farming, but it's hard when Mother Nature takes an animal when you're not looking. I know it seems odd, but this is how farming works: We work our butts off keeping animals alive and healthy, then we kill them.

Domestic livestock can be attacked by predators: coyotes and wolves, foxes and eagles, packs of dogs running together. Hawks and other small birds of prey can pick off a chicken or small duck before you can blink.

Animals can also die as a result of accidents, or from injuries they cause one another. Our favorite goat, Pokey, started as a little black-and-white-polka-dotted guy and grew into a magnificent and friendly beast. He lived for several years in the barn with the rams, Jeffrey and Duncan, and he was a happy guy. One day we needed to lock the three of them up for a few hours in a good-sized pen so that we could do some fence work in their enclosure. For some reason, this ticked off Jeffrey and he took it out on Pokey.

At least that's what we were able to piece together. By the time Melissa let the boys out, Pokey was oddly subdued and within hours was shaking uncontrollably. He went downhill from there. Melissa tried everything she knew; she called the vet and asked for advice, gave Pokey shots, but nothing worked. Three days later Melissa went up to the barn and found Pokey on the ground, dead.

A postmortem revealed massive internal bleeding caused by a traumatic injury. The only way he could have been injured like that was if Jeffrey had rammed him hard, really hard. In some sort of weird testosterone thing, Jeffrey killed his playmate. Other farmers tell stories of rams killing other rams, of cows beating up on each other. These aren't animals in confinement; these are animals with plenty of room. Sometimes animals can be nasty. Chickens will peck another to death if they sense weakness, or if they see a spot of blood already on the poor hen's feathers.

Even in sustainable farming systems, it can be a challenge keeping animals alive so that they can fulfill their purpose. Is it wrong, in the grand scheme of life, to assign a purpose to an animal's life? Philosophers and animal rights activists may debate this all they want, but I must consider purpose in the context of my life. As a farmer, using agricultural land productively to feed people, my animals have a purpose: to produce offspring that will become meat, or to become meat themselves.

The days on which we deliver animals to the processor certainly aren't easy, but I don't have a problem with the idea that animals must be killed. If I did, I wouldn't still be in this business, and I wouldn't still be eating meat. It's *how* most animals are killed, however, that disturbs me.

# A Disassembly
# Line

••• ••• •••••• ••• •••

*ABATTOIR* IS SUCH a lovely word to say, rolling off the tongue much like *boudoir, armoire, Guy Noir.* Yet an abattoir isn't, by nature, a lovely place. To have animals killed, the farmer takes them to an abattoir, also called a slaughterhouse, a meatpacking plant, an animal processing plant. Call it whatever you want, it's where an animal makes that transition from animal to meat. The word *abattoir* comes from the French verb *abattre,* which means "to strike down."

Just as farms have grown into factories, small, careful abattoirs have grown into gigantic disassembly lines. Until our population shifted from rural to urban in the twentieth century, many people killed their own meat, so the death of animals was visible to all. It still is in many countries. Richard Bulliet writes in *Hunters, Herders, and Hamburgers* that a 2004 show of hands in a Beirut University class indicated that 90 percent of the students had witnessed animal slaughter, compared to well under 20 percent at Columbia University in New York City.[2]

As I've mentioned, I'm not wild about killing my own meat. But because for years I've let corporations do it for me without paying attention, keeping me a happily stuffed little bird, those same corporations have gone wild with the widget thing. They not only strive to raise more animals on a piece of land or in a building, but they also strive to kill more animals per day in their processing plants.

According to the 1958 Humane Slaughter Act, "No method of slaughtering or handling in connection with slaughtering shall be deemed to comply with the public policy of the United States unless it is humane." The definition of humane is that all livestock "are rendered insensible to pain by a single blow or gunshot or an electrical, chemical or other means that is rapid and effective, before being shackled, hoisted, thrown, cast or cut."[3]

If the United States had the money to put enough inspectors in every plant, we might have been able to ensure that the law was followed. It hasn't been.

Here's how it's supposed to work. Ideally, the animal will be moved calmly and without stress into the handling facility, which funnels the animals down to single file, where they are restrained in a stanchion. The employee called a knocker renders the animal unconscious. The catcher attaches a shackle to one of the animal's rear legs, and the animal is hoisted up and begins moving along a conveyor line. The sticker slices through the carotid artery, and the animal bleeds out and dies. Skinners remove the hide, the head, and the intestines. The animal is cut in two lengthwise (here's where the term "side of beef" came from), then cut up and packaged for shipment.

What goes wrong? Not every animal is successfully stunned, which means an animal may end up hanging by its back leg, terrified and kicking. The sticker's job suddenly becomes very dangerous, and he may not do it successfully, so the animal continues, dazed but alive, farther down the line. You get the picture.

*Yoga Journal* describes what can happen: "USDA regulates the maximum speeds of livestock processing assembly lines, but the speeds can be as fast as 390 cows and 1106 pigs per hour, and 25 chickens per minute. If line workers fail to keep up with those speeds, they risk being disciplined or fined . . . the high quotas mean that workers often resort to violent measures to keep the lines running, dismembering or skinning animals that are still struggling and kicking."[4]

The USDA disagrees. A spokesperson said, "We have inspectors in every plant, and if it did occur [live animals moving down the line], that would be unacceptable."

Eric Schlosser wrote in *Mother Jones*: "The golden rule in meatpacking plants is 'The Chain Will Not Stop.' USDA inspectors can shut down the line to ensure food safety, but the meatpacking firms do everything possible to keep it moving at top speed. Nothing stands in the way of production, not mechanical failures, breakdowns, accidents. Forklifts crash, saws overheat, workers drop knives, workers get cut, workers collapse and lie unconscious on the floor, as dripping carcasses sway past them, and the chain keeps going."[5]

This brings up an externality of factory butchering—the impact on the employees in those plants. Schlosser writes that thirty years ago meatpacking was one of the highest-paid industrial jobs in the United States and had very low employee turnover rates. "Meatpacking jobs were dangerous and unpleasant, but provided enough income for a solid, middle-class life. There were sometimes waiting lists for these jobs."

No more. The model has changed to low skill and low wage. Wages have fallen by 50 percent. The turnover rate is 100 percent, which means the plants replace their entire workforce every year, which in turn means few workers acquire the skills necessary to do the job correctly. To make matters worse, twenty-five years ago the speed of the beef slaughtering line was 175 animals an hour. Now it's up to 400.[6]

According to the Bureau of Labor Statistics, meatpacking is this country's most dangerous occupation. Schlosser listed titles from accident reports filed by the Occupational Safety and Health Administration, and they provide a frightening sampling of the externalities slaughterhouse workers pay for killing our meat: Employee Hospitalized for Neck Laceration from Flying Blade. Employee's Finger Amputated in Sausage Extruder. Employee's Eye Injured When Struck by Hanging Hook. Employee's Arm Amputated in Meat Auger. Employee Killed When Head Crushed in Hide Fleshing Machine. Employee Killed by Stun Gun. I could go on, but you get the picture.

I am so grateful that another person kills the animals for me that I think we should have a national day of gratitude where we gather outside the nearest meatpacking plant and shake the hand of every person coming off shift. Or instead we could let the corporations know we will no longer support the torture of both animals and humans with our meat dollars.

The largest slaughterhouse in the world is the Smithfield Packing Company in Smithfield, Virginia, capable of butchering more than thirty thousand pigs a day. Other hog abattoirs might process seven thousand animals a day. Plants in Kansas and Colorado disassemble sixty-four hundred steers per day.

Some animals come in with manure already on their hides. In the high-speed disassembly world, the hides may come in contact with the meat itself and contaminate the meat—think E. coli. And if an animal makes it to the conveyor line still alive, it'll be terrified and evacuate its bowels—think more E. coli.

The current governmental regulations on slaughterhouses apply only to mammals. Poultry in large slaughterhouses do not have to be stunned before being killed, so they can be treated as if they are dead before they actually are dead. When the chicken crates arrive at the plant, they are tipped over, and the chickens tumble down a ramp that "resembles a playground slide."[7] All animals are terrified when they fall down and are frantic to get up again, since falling makes animals feel vulnerable to attack.

The chickens' legs are attached to a moving chain overhead, they're dunked in a tank of electrified water to stun them, then they're moved along, hopefully by now unconscious, to where a blade cuts off their head. The problem isn't the killing; the problem is the automated part of it. Animals are not always rendered unconscious, so they struggle and evade the blade, and might make it far down the disassembly line still alive. There are plants in Missouri that kill and process three hundred thousand chickens per day, which is more than three hundred chickens every minute. Try doing *anything* with animals this quickly, and things will go very wrong.

Author Rod Dreher quotes a state chicken inspector at a small processing plant: "If I were at a high-volume poultry processing plant instead of here today, I would be looking at 15,000 chickens instead of your 200. . . . No way you can look at 15,000 chickens in eight hours of work and properly evaluate the quality of that meat."[8]

Even though I'm a carnivore, this is not what I signed up for. During my thirty years of adulthood, as I worked hard in school and at my jobs and on the farm, I paid grocery stores and restaurants to feed me. But as I did this, I didn't intend to send the message that I didn't care what happened to my meat before it hit my plate. This, however, is the message I've been sending. It's not okay with me that animals are still conscious when they are hung by their legs and cut up. It's not okay with me that live chickens are tumbled down a slide, especially when there are other options. For example, a large plant in Nebraska uses a "modern controlled atmosphere stunning method." Basically, they flood a compartment with a gas that renders the chickens unconscious, a much more effective and humane practice than *not* stunning them.

The Humane Society of the United States has been challenging the USDA on its exclusion of poultry from the Humane Methods of Slaughter Act. In the United Kingdom an organization called the Humane Slaughter Association is "committed to the welfare of animals in markets, during transport and to the point of slaughter," and hopes to make "a lasting and practical improvement to the welfare of food animals."[9] A few more chicken processing plants have begun using gas, and in March 2007 Burger King announced it would begin favoring suppliers of chicken who use this method over electric shock.[10]

Temple Grandin has worked very hard to improve the conditions in U.S. slaughterhouses. Her favorite animal is the cow, so she's been motivated to ease their fears as much as possible. What gets an animal's heart racing are things they don't understand, like sparkling reflections on puddles of water, metal clanging or banging, jiggling chains, blowing air, a piece of clothing hung over a fence, drain grates on floors, entering a dark place, or seeing people move up ahead. Thanks to Grandin, most of the major slaughterhouses now use handling facilities designed to ease animals' fears and move them more quickly from pens into the abattoir. She designed pens and corrals that calm animals; they can't see what's around them, but just focus on the animal in front of them.

Grandin also has designed tools the plants can use to make sure they are doing a good job. Unfortunately, not everyone takes her advice. Government regulators come up with one-hundred-point audits for analyzing a plant, which tend to focus inspectors' attention on fussy details like measuring the floor grates, examining worker training schedules, or plant maintenance procedures.

They also usually go for a zero-tolerance approach, which on the surface sounds great: make sure no animal ever gets hurt. The problem is, that's almost impossible to achieve, given the number of animals and workers and the nature of the process. So if a plant makes a mistake, it gets shut down, the employees are out of work, there's a big stink, and management pressures the inspector to alter the report so that everyone can get back to work.

Grandin argues there's a better way to protect animals: "People can live up to high standards, but they can't live up to perfection. When you give a plant a good standard—like 95 percent of all cattle have to be stunned (killed) correctly on the first shot every single day—they always do better than they do under zero-tolerance regulation."[11]

Of course, this approach isn't perfect, because if a million cattle are slaughtered in a day, 5 percent of this amount is fifty thousand animals. Do I like the idea that fifty thousand animals might be mistreated as they are killed? No, but in Grandin's opinion, and in mine, this is much better than what happens in plants with zero tolerance, where violations are ignored and change never happens.

Instead of that list of one hundred points, where violating one item becomes minor because there are so many, Grandin came up with five key measurements inspectors can use to ensure animals receive humane treatment at a meatpacking plant. Violating one of them is a huge thing, since there are so few points. To be more humane, Grandin wants a plant to accomplish these five goals:

1. 95 percent of the animals should be stunned, or killed, correctly on the first attempt.
2. 100 percent of the animals must remain unconscious after stunning.
3. No more than three out of every one hundred animals should vocalize during handling. If an animal is calm,

it won't say anything. But if you have an animal bellowing, there's something wrong.
4. No more than one out of one hundred animals should
ever fall down.
5. Employees should use the electric prod on no more
than 25 percent of the animals for an acceptable score,
or no more than 5 percent for an excellent score. The
prod is necessary because Holsteins often balk at moving forward.[12]

In addition, Grandin came up with a list of five behaviors that
will result in an automatic failure of the plant's audit: (1) drag-
ging a live animal with a chain, (2) running cattle on top of one
another on purpose, (3) sticking prods or other objects into sensitive parts of animals, (4) purposely slamming gates on animals,
and (5) losing control and beating an animal.[13] Add these five to
the five goals earlier, and Grandin's ten things that *shouldn't* happen in a plant show me an uncomfortably accurate picture of
what *does* happen.

Grandin's guidelines are having some effect. In 1999 McDonald's started auditing the plants that supplied them with meat
and threw a major plant off the approved supplier list for flunk-
ing the audit, and they suspended some other plants. As Grandin
writes, "Let me tell you, you go out there now and they're handling the cattle *nice*. All of the plants being audited using my list
treat their animals better than plants using 100-item checklists.
Most large plants are now audited by restaurant chains like Mc-
Donald's, Burger King, and Wendy's."[14]

These changes are just a drop in the bucket. The most vocal
voices, the ones who can roar loudly enough to be heard, are the
people on whose behalf all of this slaughter is taking place: us. If
we don't use our meat dollars to support more humane slaughter,
little will change.

# Letter to
# My Lambs

··· ··· ······ ··· ···

WELL, LAMBIES, THE time has come. We called Doug and he'll be arriving at 6:00 A.M. tomorrow with his trailer to pick you up.

You're not going to like the trailer because you've never been in one before. To get you to jump up inside, I'll likely have to lead you with a bucket of corn. Once inside, you'll relax, though, because you're with your buddies.

It's a short ride to the abattoir, and some of you might even relax enough to lie down and chew your cud. Melissa will be sitting ahead of you in the cab of the pickup truck; it's important for her to be with you every step of the way—up until that last step, anyway. I'll be at my desk writing, but my thoughts will be following you all the way down there.

I just wanted to let you know how much I've loved you these last nine months. I know you don't think about the past and the future, but it's been a joy watching you grow. When you were born, your ears were much too large for your face, so you looked as if you were wearing windmills. If you were sleeping or looking the other way, I could come behind you and pick you up. Your heart raced, of course, but after a few minutes you'd relax and let me inhale your babiness, your warm, tightly curled wool, and stroke your fuzzy ears.

After a few weeks your body filled out and you became round and firm, and with that firmness came a new courage to explore. You and your buddies loved to race up and down the pasture, often without parental permission, going off for hours at a time, likely giving your moms a few more gray fibers in their wool.

Before I could even blink, you were teenagers, and suddenly it was all about the food. Eat, eat, eat was all you wanted to do. You still nursed from your mother, but sometimes you would bash her bag so fiercely to let the milk down that her back end would rise nearly a foot off the ground. We let you stay with your mom until she grew tired of the bashing and weaned you by simply walking away whenever you tried to nurse. She was still there for you, of course, because every night you'd leave your buddies and tuck in close beside your mom and siblings.

When we finally separated you from your mothers, we knew we'd done the right thing waiting until your mamas had weaned you, because most of you hardly noticed, too excited to be moving to fresh pasture. A few of you mama's boys cried a bit for a day or two, but then seemed to settle into your new independence quickly.

So now, after all these months of your eating grass, hay, and corn, I can barely recognize the fragile little lambs in you. You're all big bruisers, and at least one of you has come up behind me and rammed my butt and then melted into the crowd, all innocence when I whirled around to confront you.

Sending you off to the butcher is not an easy thing. Your presence on our farm has so enriched my life.

I know there are many people in this world who think I'm cruel to raise you and then condemn you to the slaughterhouse to be someone's meal. Some people think it's wrong to eat meat, and I respect their right to have that opinion. But if the world stopped eating meat, we'd see fewer and fewer of you. No offense, but you can't survive on your own. Your wild cousins can, but you can't. All it would take is a few months in the wild, and the coyotes, wolves, feral dogs, and eagles would kill most of you.

A few of you might live on in zoos or state fair petting zoos. Some hobby farmers with money to burn might be willing to have you around for pastoral atmosphere, but you cost so much to feed, and require so much energy to keep safe and healthy, that few farmers could afford to have you around just because you're cute. And unless people suddenly want to start wearing more wool, I'm afraid that's not going to pay for your room and board.

I know it's selfish, but I can't imagine a world without you sheep. I would miss your cousins climbing those impossibly steep hills in Scotland and northern England. I would miss seeing small farm flocks as I drive through the Midwest. I would miss your presence in my life.

I know that sounds as if it's all about me, but it's not . . . it's about you and me. It's about me working with nature to harvest the sun's energy and convert it into food for humans. It's about you having a great nine months of life. It's about the two of us continuing to do what sheep and shepherds have done for more than ten thousand years, and I am deeply honored to be woven into the tapestry that reaches so far back into our past.

Tomorrow morning, when we load you onto the trailer for your trip to the abattoir, we will be thinking about the life you've lived on this farm—running around the pasture at dusk, sleeping in the sun, and grazing enthusiastically for the tenderest bits of grass. We will say out loud, "Thank you."

You will die quickly tomorrow. You won't be part of a kill and disassembly line, but you will be killed, one at a time. I'd say that

I appreciate your sacrifice, but you aren't making the choice to die. I'm making it, and I take full responsibility for that.

Your mothers are all pregnant again, and your fathers are recovering from their blissful four weeks of sex. In three months new lambs will be born, and we will begin your story all over again.

I wish you a safe journey, and I honor your role in my life.

# Inside an
# Abattoir

••• ••• •••••• ••• •••

I VALUE ITEMS that are made by hand—hand-spun yarn, hand-knit sweaters, homemade pies and cookies instead of store-bought pies and cookies—and I've decided I feel the same way about my meat. I'd prefer meat from animals killed individually, one by one, rather than killed on a disassembly line. Small farmers who finish their animals for processing use small abattoirs. It's a different experience because these smaller facilities aren't set up with a huge production line. Each animal is, for a brief moment, the only thing the employee focuses on. Great care is taken not to let feces and meat mingle.

Chickens are taken from their cages, one by one, and placed upside-down in plastic cones with their heads poking out the bottom. Most chickens will be calm when this happens. When an employee cuts the chicken's main artery, the chicken loses consciousness, bleeds out, and dies. Every animal is attended to by hand and will not be processed further until it has died. No terrifying slides, no live chickens hung up by their legs. It's over very quickly.

For years we took our sheep to a family-owned abattoir only fifteen minutes from our farm. This meant the sheep had a very short trip, minimizing their stress. When we delivered our sheep to this plant, we'd back up the trailer to a high-sided set of metal panels, one of those handling facilities Temple Grandin designed. The system funneled the animals single file into a chute leading to the kill floor. Here's the part where courageous me hopped into the truck and drove away, or perhaps stepped into the pristine white hallway leading to the offices to discuss our customers' orders.

The one place I haven't gone in this small abattoir is the other direction, down the long, white hallway and up a narrow staircase enclosed by concrete block walls. At the top of the stairs is a small viewing area. If I turn to the right, I will be looking through a massive plate-glass window down into the kill floor. If I turn left, I will be looking down into the cutting room.

I've seen the cutting room, and even spent a day there helping a man create some experimental lamb products. Employees wear white coats, white pants, and hairnets. One works at a massive saw cutting steaks. Another feeds meat into a grinder to make hamburger. Another wheels a rack of bacon out of the smokehouse in the corner, releasing such incredible scents my mouth waters just writing about it. Few carnivores would have trouble watching the activity in this room; in fact, it's very interesting to watch the machine that makes sausage, to watch the automatic packaging machine, to see how efficiently meat is prepared for us.

It's getting harder and harder for small farmers to find abattoirs. The place we worked with grew larger and could no longer make money by processing sheep. We found another abattoir nearby, but the people there didn't have much experience cutting lamb.

We have finally found a great plant that works well for us. When Melissa delivered the first twenty lambs to this facility, she asked them to explain how the animals would be killed. Regulations have changed, and unlike the methods used by our previous processors, animals are no longer shot in the head to be stunned, but are instead given an electric shock. An employee showed her a device with a Y-shaped prong that fits behind the sheep's head. One jolt and the animal is unconscious.

What next? The animal's back legs are attached to chains and hydraulically raised off the ground, but in this particular plant there is no conveyor line. Other small plants may be large enough to have lines, but their kill rate is going to be slower than the mega-disassembly lines. As the unconscious animal hangs there, the butcher cuts its throat, after which it bleeds out and dies.

The feet and hide then come off, or in the case of hogs, the carcass is dipped in hot water and the hair removed. Then everything inside the carcass must come out—internal organs, rumen, intestines, anus, and so forth. Somewhere in the process the head comes off and is set aside. Unless the internal organs and head and hide are going to be used, they are considered waste products, or offal, and are trucked away to be composted, or sold to a company that will convert the waste material into something useful. Thankfully, very little of the inedible material goes to waste. According to the American Beef Council, 99 percent of every steer butchered is used.[15] Beef by-products show up in candles, crayons, cosmetics, detergent, insulation, plastics, soaps, pet foods, piano keys, luggage, wallpaper, camera film, insulin, car polish, and textiles for auto upholstery. The list for hog and sheep by-products is similar.

With the head and feet and hide gone, an animal has made the visual transition from animal to meat and is now a carcass hanging by a hook in a cooler. How long a carcass hangs depends on the butcher—beef might hang for a week to allow the chemical composition of the muscles to change and become more palatable. Lamb carcasses can be easily cut the next day.

Carcasses are cut up with saws; some parts are ground into burger, and others are put into sausage. The meat is wrapped by a machine, weighed, labeled, and frozen.

We learned the hard way that animal stress makes a difference in the quality of the meat itself. Even in a small processing plant things can go wrong. Several years ago a lamb customer got up the courage to tell us that that year's meat was very tough, almost inedible. We were horrified, of course, so we checked with a few other customers. Two others confessed their lamb was too tough to eat; a few more said theirs was fine. We offered to replace the tough lamb, and I retrieved some of the meat so we could try it ourselves, knowing that lamb can become tough if you cook it too long.

No, it wasn't a cooking problem. The meat was horrible, and we were terribly confused. All the animals in that year's crop had eaten the same grass and legumes all summer long. All had eaten the same corn, the same hay during the winter months. They were all healthy when we took them to the abattoir. What could have gone wrong?

Then Melissa remembered the butchering day. With an employee's help, she had unloaded our lambs early that morning, then stepped outside to shut a gate. When she got back inside, the employee, obviously having a bad day, was cursing and smacking the animals nearest him with a huge paddle, frustrated because they weren't moving forward. Sheep won't move when treated that way. Horrified, Melissa stopped him, moved the animals into the correct pen herself, and then reported the abuse. If an animal is under great stress, its muscle composition changes temporarily; if butchered during this time, the muscles stay tense and the meat is tough. Our theory is that the customers who received tough meat received the animals that the man had been hitting.

We weren't just imagining this. *The Grassfed Gourmet* explains what happens: "Animals that are stressed at slaughter will secrete surplus adrenaline and lactic acid, causing the meat to be tough and to have an off-flavor."[16]

We replaced a few orders but stopped there, unable financially to replace everyone's order. The next year approximately 25 percent of the customers did not order from us again. How an animal is treated, and how an animal is killed, is not just an ethical issue, but an economic one as well.

Sometimes the most humane butchers are those who truly understand how to kill and process an animal. Many people in society used to think hunters were horrible people who tracked down Bambi, killed, and ate him. Some still think this. I don't, since most of the hunters I know are doing it not just as a sport but also to feed their families. Besides, I fail to see how we non-hunters can take the moral high ground when we are paying factories to raise an animal in confinement like a widget and kill it as part of a disassembly line. How is that any more compassionate than a hunter killing an animal that has lived a totally free and natural life?

Hunters, and farmers who raise and butcher their own animals, understand how important it is to kill and process an animal in the most humane way. As written in *Basic Butchering of Livestock and Game:* "The animal must be killed quickly, with little or no pain, but more important is that death comes without fear. To allow an animal to become frightened at slaughter is not only cruel, but unwise, for it causes the release of adrenaline, which some believe can affect the quality of the meat. Also, fear may cause the animal to struggle, doing damage to its meat or injuring the person slaughtering."[17]

We need a clear-eyed view of farming, one that doesn't romanticize sustainable farms as animal sanctuaries. Farms raise livestock animals for people to consume, and this is true whether the farm is a massive CAFO, a midsize conventional farm, or a small organic farm. Roger Scruton successfully captures the realities of raising animals for meat:

> There's a real distinction for a human being, between timely and untimely death. To be "cut short" before one's time is a waste— even a tragedy. . . . No such thoughts apply to domestic cattle. To be killed at thirty months is not intrinsically more tragic than to be killed at forty, fifty or sixty. And if the meat is at its best after thirty months . . . who will blame a farmer for choosing so early a death? In doing so he merely reflects the choice of the consumer, upon whose desires the whole trade in meat, and therefore the very existence of his animals, depends.[18]

The lives of animals on sustainable or small farms are not necessarily all that much longer than in a factory; the difference is quality, not quantity. If we let every animal on our farm grow old instead of heading for the food supply, we'd go broke running a dude ranch or animal sanctuary. For years on this farm, when we determined an animal was no longer productive, we sold it at the livestock market.

Of course, if after twelve years we find ourselves softening a bit when it comes to a handful of really old ewes who've given us twins every year and been great mothers, but who now have bad udders or are too old to breed, and we decide to let those animals remain on the farm until they die, we certainly wouldn't tell anyone, and I certainly wouldn't admit that in a book.

••• ••• •••

For many years Melissa had no problems standing in the abattoir watching another farmer's animals killed, but wasn't ready to see this happen to one of our own. This year, however, she was ready. A friend, an experienced hunter and former farm boy, wanted to buy a lamb and slaughter it himself. One frosty February morning he and Melissa met behind our sheep barn, and Melissa pointed to the large lamb she'd picked out the night before. Together, they held the lamb by his tail and his head, the standard method for walking a sheep forward, and gently walked him out of the pen to the butcher site. The lamb was irritated at being directed like that, but not terrified. Then, before the lamb knew what was happening, our friend put a gun at the base of the animal's skull and shot it. Melissa said the animal lost consciousness and crumpled to the ground, bleeding profusely. The animal's death was very, very quick.

The next time Melissa took our animals to the abattoir, she decided to hang around and watch. Once again, the process was quick, calm, and respectful. The animal was moved into a small restraining pen and the back of its head soaked with water, since wool can interfere with the shocker. Then the guy positioned the electric Y-pronged shocker at the base of the animal's skull and pushed the button. The animal dropped, instantly unconscious.

The employee hooked a chain onto one back leg, and the animal was lifted by a hydraulic block and tackle into the air, still unconscious. The man, using a very sharp knife and possessing the skill to know just where to put that knife, cut off the head. Blood gushed down onto the floor. When the blood stopped, he attached an automatic skinner, which slowly peeled the skin off, revealing the animal's layer of fat around its muscles. The chest cavity was cut open, and the intestines removed. An inspector checked the head, the intestines, and the carcass itself for problems, but saw none.

I tend to get squeamish when someone tries to explain to me how veins and arteries work, but Melissa finds the inner workings of animals fascinating. Watching an animal being taken apart is always a learning experience for her, and she has no problems with it, as long as the animal isn't one she's known for a long time. She will not be watching our steer being slaughtered.

Although thinking about the trillions of animals being raised in factories makes me angry, thinking about those same animals being killed with so little respect and consideration actually hurts my heart. It's wrong, wrong, wrong. Both carnivores and animal rights/welfare groups are finally getting on the same page: regardless of how one feels about eating animals, no one wants to see them suffer. When I spend my money on meat raised by a factory, I'm paying that factory not only to continue raising more animals that way, but also to continue killing them in a manner that harms us all.

I don't know about you, but I find that focusing so intently on killing animals is hard work. I need a break. I need to spend some time with my animals, with some *live* animals.

Part Six

# Time for a Break: Taking a Pasture Walk

How beautiful it is to do nothing,
and then rest afterward.

—SPANISH PROVERB

Time slows down on a pasture walk. On a pasture walk you won't find tips or self-help suggestions or facts. You won't find anything to do with buying meat or making choices or changing your meat-eating habits. You'll find fresh air, animals, and perhaps a bit of peace. At least that's what I experience on a pasture walk. You might also come away with a greater appreciation for the animals. Appreciating them doesn't mean you can't eat them; it just means your level of respect, concern, and compassion for animals' lives might increase.

So put on some sturdy shoes—no sandals or heels—because pastures can be notoriously uneven ground, especially ours. Wear pants so the knee-high grass won't tickle your legs, and to discourage wood ticks from using your leg as a blood bank.

A hat against the hot Minnesota sun (don't laugh, July and August can be beastly) wouldn't be a bad thing, although I like to stick to the shade as much as possible.

There's nothing like plopping down under a thick canopy of branches, taking care not to sit in any recently deposited manure, then grabbing a stem of tender grass to tear apart or wind around your fingers as we talk. When there's a refreshing breeze sweeping over us and birds are twittering overhead with a background chorus of crickets, everything falls away—bills, jobs, health problems, conflict. Breathe deeply, then join me on a meandering walk through the pasture.

# Talking to
# Animals

••• ••• •••••• ••• •••

FOR MOST OF my life, my understanding of domestic farm animals came from observing them from the corners of my eyes as I sped by at seventy miles an hour. I actually thought that sheep did nothing more than stand in one place and graze. I assumed, of course, that they would walk now and then, perhaps moving from pasture to barn, but I didn't imagine they would do more than that.

It wasn't until I started farming that I realized animals weren't just inanimate props stuck out in a pasture so photographers could capture a romantic pastoral scene. They weren't just standing around waiting to be butchered. They run, play, and fight.

Animals communicate with one another. A ewe and her lambs each have unique voices that help them find each other in a crowd. When we move the entire flock from one paddock to the next for fresh grass, the family groups get all mixed up, so once they're in the new place a cacophony of bleats rises up. It's amazing to watch the mothers and babies find each other by calling. Two lambs standing together each cry, the ewe answers, the lambs move in her direction through the crowd, cry again, the ewe answers. Eventually the lambs get close enough to recognize Mom, race toward her, and drink for all they're worth, their wagging tails saying, "Boy, we thought we'd lost you!" Nothing is sweeter than the silence after a ewe and her lambs have reunited.

Animals communicate with us. If we leave the flock in a particular paddock a day longer than we should, the good grass is gone and the sheep have peed or pooped on what's left. When Melissa or I show up, perhaps not intending to move them but to check on them, the sheep run for us, then stand there bellowing indignantly. Even if I'm pressed for time, the guilt is enough to get me off the four-wheeler to set up the fences and move them into fresh grass. The sheep have learned that bellowing indignantly is an effective communication technique.

The only time it doesn't work is in the fall. In Minnesota the grass usually stops growing around mid-October. After the sheep spend a few weeks eating what's left, we have no choice but to bring them back to the barn and start feeding them hay. Hay has the nutrition and fiber they need, but it just doesn't taste as good as fresh, plump blades of grass. It's like people switching from fresh, succulent corn on the cob to dehydrated corn.

The sheep make no bones about not liking hay. They yell at us for a few weeks, but since we don't do anything about this nasty dry food we've given them, they eventually give up and settle in for a few months of eating it.

If the sheep are frightened by something I'm doing, like, say, *chasing* them, they run away. This is a form of communication. It's also the method we use to make the sheep go where they need to go.

Animals communicate what's going on in the pasture. We heard a presentation the other day on protecting your flock from wolves and coyotes, and the shepherd speaking urged us all to watch our flocks' behavior. If the animals are flighty when a farmer shows up, running suddenly, or just not settling down to chew cud, that flock has likely been visited the night before by a predator, and they're still spooked.

Llamas communicate by watching. If I look out my kitchen window and all three llamas are looking to the east, that means there is a strange animal to the east. Perhaps it's a fox, a coyote, or just a deer innocently passing through the pasture; it's good to know, and might be worth investigating.

If you were to walk into one of our pastures without us (not recommended, by the way), the llama in charge will come right up to you. In doing so, he's sending you a message: "Back away from the sheep and no one will get hurt." Just his size alone should be enough to encourage you to back up and leave. I once took some friends out to the pasture to meet our llama Chachi, but when he approached, I was suddenly all alone. My friends had lined up behind me in some imagined safety zone.

Anyone fleeing the law out in the country should avoid hiding in pastures or lots with cattle, since the cattle will gather around the new guy and stare, a dead giveaway to the farmer that something, or someone, is out there.

Just as humans are more likely to hang out with friends instead of strangers, animals feel that same connection to other animals they know. Temple Grandin tells an amazing story about how animals use that sociability to communicate. At one particularly huge livestock auction, truck after truck of hogs was unloaded by the livestock market employees. Confusingly, each truck ended up a few hogs short of the number claimed to be on board. Obviously someone was stealing a pig or two off of each load. But who? And where were those pigs going?

The pigs from each truck were kept in separate pens, and after a few days workers noticed that in one pen the pigs were keeping their distance from one another, acting like strangers. That was because they *were* strangers—they'd all come from different farms and didn't know each other. An employee had been stealing a hog from each truck and sticking the animal into this pen, thinking no one would notice.

The pigs noticed. And because one of the stockyard workers understood pig communication, he was able to hear what they were saying: "Hey, these pigs aren't my friends. They smell funny. They look funny. I don't belong with these pigs!"[1]

One of the joys of being a small farmer is that we can take the time to communicate with, and observe, our animals. After spending thirty minutes standing in the pasture, Melissa will know which ewe might be feeling a bit under the weather, which one might be angry at another sheep, which ewe might have a sore udder.

I obviously don't believe this intense and enriching communication means we can't eat these animals; it means we feel closer to them, and even more committed to making sure we take good care of them while they are here on this farm, on this earth.

Some people take the idea of communication very literally and believe they can have actual conversations with animals. I suppose this sort of communication with your pets would be pretty cool. But to try to communicate on this level with your meat? Hmmm, maybe not.

It seems like the perfect recipe for disaster. What if you find out way more than you want to know? What if you find out so much that you can't actually keep farming? What if you actually connect on such a level that you walk around the farm hearing the animals expressing their opinions and wry observations night and day? This is why I was stunned the day Melissa announced she was interested in learning more about animal communication.

"Why?" I asked. "What if you're able to communicate with a hen and she says, 'Please stop stealing my children and scrambling them and putting them in quiches'? What if a ewe says,

'That needle hurts. Please don't give me a shot.' Or, god forbid, what if a lamb, on the way to the abattoir, says, 'Where are we going?'"

No, no, no. Not a good idea.

But something about the idea of reaching an animal's mind fascinated Melissa, and because animals are such a huge part of her life, to be offered the chance to connect on an even deeper level was too compelling to pass up.

So despite my pleas, she and our dog Sophie attended the Animal Communication Workshop a few hours' drive north. I sullenly did chores and worried.

It turns out that the idea of animal communication isn't quite as literal as I'd thought. Apparently most people can't just sit down and chat over tea and doggie biscuits with animals. While there are some superintuitive people who maintain they can communicate directly, most of us must be content with something more elusive.

"It's a matter of sending images in your mind," Melissa said when she returned, still interested but less than enthusiastic, since apparently Sophie hadn't received any of the images. "Animals aren't verbal," Melissa continued, "so instead you're supposed to create an image in your mind of what you want them to know or do, and keep sending this image over and over again."

After a few more workshops, Melissa conceded that she was too scientific to believe in the whole idea and gave up. But we did find that when desperate we would try it anyway, sending images of good behavior to whatever animal was doing something naughty.

One year during shearing, about fifteen sheared ewes were out by the hay bales with Chachi, our oldest llama. I wasn't paying any attention to them, since we were all focused on the activity of shearing, gathering up the wool, and listening to our shearer tell stories. At one point my mom, who'd brought the day's food, touched my arm and pointed to Chachi. "Is he supposed to be doing that?"

Chachi was running the sheep up to the barn, then back out to the hay bales, then back up to the barn. It was unnecessary, and probably not the best idea for pregnant sheep to be running their own 5K. So I tramped all the way out to the hay bales, not quite sure how to make this guy stop his fun. When I reached Mr. Tall, Dark, and Handsome, I just started talking, telling him it really wasn't necessary to make the sheep run back and forth. No sign of understanding filled those luminous black eyes, so I clutched at the only straw I had: images. I bombarded the guy with images of him cushing, which is what llamas do when they fold up their legs and sit on them. Images of the sheep lying down. Images of Chachi cushing, cushing, sitting there not running the sheep. Finally, all imaged-out, I turned my back on Chachi and marched back up to the barn, where my mother waited. Only when I reached her did I turn around. Back at the bales, Chachi—I swear this to be true—was cushing.

I explained my animal communication to my mom. "I don't know whether to be really impressed," she said, "or really frightened."

None of my attempts since has worked, but I still send images, usually when I'm tired of chasing an animal and am desperate. I've learned, however, that before I move the sheep it works much better to stop and consider the animal's world. If I were a sheep, what would I do if a human approached? Where would I go? What would frighten me and how could I be safe? That's the animal communication that works best for me.

So while I do talk to my animals, they don't talk back, which is a relief, since talking animals belong in movies and books, not reality. But I find that if I pay attention, my animals do have plenty to say.

# Do Sheep
# Feel Sheepish?

···  ···  ······  ···  ···

FIGURING OUT ANIMALS' personalities can be an exacting science. Scientists have found that the cute whorls on a cow's head may predict her disposition, since the whorl develops from the same layer of cells as the nervous system.[2] Cows with no whorl, or with a whorl above the eyes, are likely to be flighty and excitable. Drop that whorl below the eyes, and you've got a calmer cow. I'm sure this means there are livestock breeders out there trying to selectively breed for low-whorl cows.

Livestock animals feel emotions, but the range of emotions a livestock animal can actually express is more limited than, say, a dog. On many occasions I've seen our border collie look positively sheepish, but I've never in twelve years seen a sheep look sheepish. Sheep look calm, relaxed, worried, frightened, angry, and playful.

Witness baby lambs. Newborn lambs stick pretty close to Mama, but once they're a few weeks old, they're the equivalent of irrepressible human six-year-olds. Go, go, go. Those first few years we farmed, exhaustion would weigh me down, and I often wondered why the heck I was still on the farm.

Dusk became one of those reasons, my reward for the anxieties of lambing. Every summer evening around 7:00, the rowdier babies formed a gang, racing back and forth across the pasture. One evening as I watched, the gang hopped from family group to family group, enticing the more timid lambs to join them. Soon forty lambs had joined the gang, leaving only the very young lambs remaining with their mothers, watching with half envy, half alarm, as the older lambs romped.

The gang raced to the end of the paddock, then screeched to a halt, eyes wide, tiny chests heaving. One lamb leaped straight up into the air, then another, then another, as if lifted off their feet by tiny explosions. Then one lamb whirled around and began racing back. The flock of babies flowed over the ground's bumps and dips like heavy cream.

They weren't running away from anything, they weren't running to anything. They were just having a darned good time running back and forth. Maybe they were even challenging one another to see how far from their mothers they dared go. Either way, it can lighten a farmer's heart to watch her animals enjoying life.

I've had to approach ewes with newborns, and some of the bolder ewes will stand their ground until the very last minute, stamping a front foot, sometimes both, and snorting in anger.

Or when we move our sheep through the chute to give them shots or trim their hooves, we often notice that siblings, or mother and daughter, come through together. Livestock animals form attachments and recognize one another.

When the lambs are four to five months old, we separate them from the ewes, which sets a few of them bleating for a few days. It's one of the hardest things for me as a farmer to do, but there is just no way around this step, because at five months a little ram lamb is sexually ready to go. If we leave him in the same pasture as the ewes during the fall, he'll breed any ewe short enough to reach. Melissa and I learned this the hard way one year and ended up with seventeen ewes giving birth in chilly March, two months before we were ready. We wait as long as we can to wean, until the lambs are independent, but separate them we must. Everyone quiets down in a day and gets back to the serious business of eating.

Studies have shown that sheep can recognize the faces of at least ten people and fifty other sheep for at least two years. Scientists at the Babraham Institute in Cambridge also discovered that sheep react to facial expressions and, like humans, prefer a smile to a frown.[3]

Chickens can recognize up to ninety other individual chickens, which makes them much better at chicken face recognition than I am.[4] A British professor of animal husbandry, John Webster, has documented how cows within a herd form smaller groups of between two and four animals with whom they spend most of their time, often grooming and licking one another. They might also dislike other cows and can "bear grudges for months or years."[5]

Handling dairy cows with patience is a good idea. Researchers at Purdue University found that cows produced more milk if their handlers talked to them gently rather than shouting and pushing them around. A number of dairies now post signs: PLEASE DON'T SHOUT AT THE COWS.[6]

To assume animals lack emotions might make it easier for people to ignore how those animals are raised. To assume animals lack intelligence has the same result. In his book *Animal Welfare: Limping Toward Eden,* John Webster nails the relationship between intelligence and factory farming: "People have assumed that intelligence is linked to the ability to suffer and that because animals have smaller brains they suffer less than humans. That is a pathetic piece of logic."[7]

Roger Caras chimes in with a similar thought: "We have generally reckoned intelligence to be the one and only yardstick of worth. Anything less intelligent than we are—and that is everything, as we see it—deserves less, so gets less. . . . We have persistently ignored them [livestock animals] and given them what we wanted, when we wanted to, in the amounts that satisfied our needs, not theirs."[8]

I agree. While it is true most humans are smarter than animals, it is not true that this means animals don't suffer. And how do we judge an animal's intelligence?

For example, people think that sheep are dumb. If you walk among some herds of cattle, those animals may not scatter in a panic, but move slowly away. We recently toured a pasture dairy, and the herd walked right by us, not terribly concerned there were thirty strangers in their pasture. You could almost see the calves daring one another to get closer to us.

But if you walk through a flock of sheep and they don't recognize you, they'll run for the hills. If people who move cattle try moving sheep the same way you move cattle, it won't work. Sheep aren't dumb; they are just very skilled at being themselves, and not good at being cattle or hogs or dogs or people. Sheep are great at doing what is best for them—getting food and staying safe. Sheep run toward you if you have food. They run away if they think you're dangerous.

Animal and human thought processes differ because our brains differ. Temple Grandin explains that because humans make complex connections in their neocortex, we're able to experience mixed emotions—we can feel both love and hate for the same person. The animal neocortex keeps those categories more separate, so they don't experience mixed emotions.[9]

Inside the neocortex, the frontal lobes pull together all the information that's floating around in our brains. (This is why we have such attractive foreheads.) Most humans can see the big picture, but cannot see the little details that contribute to the big picture. But if something happens to a human's frontal lobe (Grandin lists head injury, developmental disabilities, or just plain old fatigue), we fall back on the animal part of our brains, which means we stop seeing the big picture, but can see the little details that animals see.[10]

Several studies have shown that domestic livestock can think and reason. Five heifers (young female cows) were trained to press a panel that would open a gate leading to food. Hidden cameras and heart rate monitors recorded the animals' physical responses. In a control group of five heifers there was no panel pushing required, and the heifers stayed calm. But in the group that had to learn to push the panel to receive food, the heifers got all excited, jumping and bucking and kicking, experiencing a sort of "eureka" moment as they enjoyed solving the problem.[11]

Another study tested hens that had been taught they would receive a small amount of food three seconds after they pecked a colored button. The smarter hens learned that if they ate the food immediately, there would be no more, but if they waited twenty-two seconds, a little Las Vegas jackpot of chicken feed would pour into the dish. The hens held out for that jackpot 90 percent of the time.[12]

In some hog farms the animals wear collars fitted with electronic receivers. When the animal approaches the entrance to the feeding area, the collar identifies the animal and a computer checks to see if the animal has already eaten its share for the day. If it has, the gate won't open for that hog and its collar. Hogs have been observed scouring the pen for another collar, one that might have come off another pig, then carrying it over to the gate, where the computer reads it, and the pig gains illegal entry for another serving of feed.[13]

Claims of anthropomorphism are often used to dismiss any attempts to ascribe emotions to animals. But while a human's personality is more complex than an animal's, and our range of emotions is wider, humans do not have exclusive rights to every emotion.

The other night at dusk I was unloading fifty-pound bags of duck feed from the back of the pickup. Calf was outside the barn watching me. When I'd walk into the barn, disappearing from his view, he'd hear me inside and run through his own door into the barn to find me dumping the bag into the feed bin. We did this twice. But before I finished pulling the third bag off the truck, the steer whirled and raced for the barn.

Know how it feels to solve a riddle or puzzle? There's that flash of excitement, that need to stand up and shout, "Hey, look what I did! I figured it out."

When I stepped inside the barn, the steer was waiting for me. All nine hundred pounds of him hopped and kicked, then he tossed his head back. I'm not anthropomorphizing to say that guy was excited. He was saying, loud and clear, *Hey, look what I did!*

I'll say this again: Acknowledging that livestock animals have personalities and emotions doesn't mean, for most of us, that we can't eat them. Instead it means we must work harder to ensure that their lives are better than they are now. Better lives mean happier animals. This is the very least we expect for the other animals in our lives—our dogs and cats—so let's raise the bar for livestock animals as well.

# Sexual Congress
## (*Between*, Not *With*, Animals)

••• ••• •••••• ••• •••

ON THIS PASTURE walk I've tried to illustrate that livestock animals communicate and that they experience emotions. I do this not to convince you to stop eating them, but to deepen your understanding of these animals and to encourage you to pay more attention to how they are raised. If we next examine the sexual activities of livestock animals, will this give you even more incentive to make changes, or give you more information for becoming a more compassionate carnivore?

Nope. When it comes to reproductive sex in livestock, there's not much difference between a large farm and a small one, or between a conventional farm and an organic one. But taking a quick peek into animals' sex lives may give you insight into the complex challenges farmers face as they produce the meat you eat. Animals are sexual beings, driven by testosterone and estrogen, which is why all farmers end up being total control freaks when it comes to animal reproduction, or there would be unauthorized sex going on all over the place.

When we started farming, it quickly became clear we had two choices for animal reproduction: let them mate naturally, or use artificial insemination. For some animals, letting them mate on their own isn't as easy as it looks. Llamas and alpacas, the smaller cousin of the llama, lie down on their bellies to reproduce, and apparently some males aren't so hot at balancing themselves while perched on the female's back. One woman sent me a photo of her partner having to kneel beside the mating alpaca pair, steadying the male so he wouldn't tip over and fall off. Heavens. How can a species survive if the male keeps tipping over mid-copulation?

Sex is all rams think about. They can smell when we've moved the ewes nearby, and they lift their heads, curling back their lips as if to drink in the Scent of Ewe. But we keep our rams and ewes separate until we're ready to have them breed—no unauthorized sheep sex on this farm. Every farmer with sexually active livestock has stories about animals violating fences—breaking down fences, jumping over fences, going through fences—just to get some action. And it's not just the rams—in the fall our ewes are as hot to trot as the boys.

When it's time to breed, we separate the ewes into two groups and put one ram in with each group. Duncan and Erik were the lucky boys this year, but because Erik is a young ram we'd never used before, we dragged out the marking harness, a clever series of straps that holds a large, rectangular marking crayon against his chest. The idea is that when the ram mounts a ewe, he'll leave a colored mark on her wool. This year we bought a green marker.

You've heard of the Scarlet Letter? On our farm this year we called it the Viridian Smudge, the mark Erik left behind on a ewe's rump to demonstrate he was doing his job. Some green smudges were big and bright green, while others weren't much more than a faint stripe. Guess he was in a hurry.

Animals, both males and females, mount animals of the same or opposite sex. The species doesn't even matter. Our steer, who weighed over five hundred pounds at the time, tried unsuccessfully to mount the rams, even though he'd been neutered. One day our ram Duncan, maybe two hundred pounds, started making goo-goo eyes at the steer, which made me laugh. The poor guy was gonna need a ladder.

On our farm we do things the old-fashioned way, letting the animals breed by themselves, albeit on our time schedule. We breed for meat quality, mothering ability, multiple births, and successful grazing. We aren't that scientific about it, but the big farms really are, studying lots of genetic traits and working to improve each one.

Sometimes breeders can reach so far for one specific trait that they breed out, or eliminate, other traits. Some of these traits, while not economically important, are very important to the animal.

Roosters come to mind. We've had some who are total gentlemen, quietly mounting a hen without ruffling anyone's feathers, the hen's or ours. We've had others who chased reluctant hens, then threw themselves on the poor squawking female.

Turns out it isn't just a personality thing, but a consequence of breeding. Chicken breeders, in a fervor to breed a "better" chicken, have messed up the roosters so badly that many roosters actually rape and kill hens.[14] Canadian researchers discovered that the rooster courtship program had been deleted in about half the roosters they studied. Apparently a normal rooster does a little courtship dance before trying to mate with a hen. Not only is this a polite thing to do, but the dance also triggers a reaction in the hen's brain that tells her to crouch down in the mating position, ready to receive the rooster. Here's the key: a hen doesn't take this position unless she sees the dance. She's hardwired that way. But since half the roosters no longer did the dance, the hens had stopped crouching for them. When a rooster mounted a hen anyway and she would try to get away, the rooster might attack her with his spurs and slash her to death.

Even if you live on a farm today, you still may not see many animals mating. Not only has modern agriculture moved animals inside, but it has also replaced natural reproduction with technology. It's more efficient to collect sperm from a male animal (now *there's* a bizarre job) and send it to farms all over the country and have vets artificially inseminate (AI) the females.

I suppose it's easier on a bull to extract his sperm than to load him on a trailer and ship him to Farm A, then Farm B, then Farm C. Animals don't really like to travel, and all that sex could wear a valuable guy out. AI is a valuable tool for improving a herd or a flock's genetics.

Getting sperm from a bull can be complex. Grandin tells the story of a Brahman bull she'd worked with who loved to be scratched and petted. He wouldn't release his semen until he'd been petted a *long* time. To impregnate the waiting cow is much easier. Insert a catheter into her womb and inject the semen. *Voilà*—pregnant cow.

And pigs? Whoa. I met a woman who worked for two months on a hog farm. Her job was to collect the boar sperm. She would release the guy into the pen, and he'd race with enthusiasm toward some sort of mechanical sow and leap aboard. The woman's job was to make sure the pig penis was properly positioned. Then once the semen was deposited into the little plastic cup, she had to smell it to make sure it smelled right, whatever that meant. And you thought your job sucked.

As Grandin wrote about collecting pig semen, "Each boar had his own little perversion the man had to do to get the boar turned on so he could collect the semen."[15] Apparently some wanted to be scratched, some wanted more . . . intimate activities.

Inseminating a cow is easy, and can apparently be done anytime. But sheep and goats must be in the correct time in their estrous cycle before they will stand willingly to be bred. Grandin said that with sows, "You have to get the sow turned on when you breed her so her uterus will pull the semen in. If she isn't fully aroused, she'll have a smaller litter because fewer eggs will get fertilized."[16] Apparently when a sow is sexually receptive, her ears pop straight up. Also, putting pressure on her back helps, because this is what she'd feel if a boar mounted her.

With sheep, we call it "standing heat," when the ewe is so ready she'll stand still for anything. I've had to move the sheep up into the barn and found one lagging behind, eventually planting herself right in front of me. "C'mon, let's go," I would urge, giving her a nudge with my knee.

Oooh. She liked that, and refused to move. The more I pushed with my knees, my legs, my shoulder, the firmer she stood, ready for a little action. I sighed, then gave up and left the ewe there, knowing I'd have one more story with which to entertain my city friends.

I joke about the sex on our farm, but I'm one of a small percentage of nonimmigrant Americans who have actually witnessed sex between animals. Richard Bulliet explored how we as a people have changed since we left the farm en masse in his book *Hunters, Herders, and Hamburgers.* He maintains that when people lived on farms and regularly witnessed "sexual congress" between animals, people had a healthier outlook on sex, because it was a natural event.[17]

I don't know if I have a healthier outlook on sex because I witness it on a much too regular basis, but I've certainly gotten used to it. When our ducks used to mate five feet from my porch swing, I'd get up and leave in disgust. Now I just mutter, "Get a room," and keep on reading.

# Part Seven

# Bowling Together
## (Slowly, Wearing an Apron)

Even if you're on the right track,
you'll get run over if you're just sitting there.

—WILL ROGERS

We've waded through the externalities associated with factory farming—the effects on the animals, on the environment, and on you. We've explored the same issues through the lens of sustainable farming. We are paying attention. We are wasting less meat.

Here's a third step to take, and it's the step that requires more thought and patience and extra effort than any of the others: Replace the factory meat in your diet with meat from animals raised humanely.

When I want to fry up an egg and there are none in the fridge, I put my barn boots on, walk out to the chicken house, and steal an egg from the nest box, which may or may not be occupied. If it's occupied, swiping that egg feels more dangerous than getting into a car and joining the seventy-mile-an-hour traffic on the highway, but I wear gloves and do it anyway.

For most of you, finding eggs from humanely raised hens is going to be a little more work than stepping outside. Try to look at it not as work, but with the same joy with which a child approaches an Easter egg hunt, where searching is just as rewarding as the prize.

There's no right or wrong way to switch from factory meat to meat from animals raised by small sustainable and organic farmers, so we each will do this in our own way. But when Melissa and I started farming, it was all new to us, and we soaked up the experience of others like sponges. What should we do first? Second? What problems would we encounter? Basically, we wanted tips on doing it better, on ensuring we would succeed. Yet we had to make our own mistakes and find our own path to becoming the farmers we wanted to be.

Just as our farming friends couldn't tell us precisely what would work on our farm, I can't tell you precisely where to find what you're looking for. I suppose I could list all the sustainable farms I could find, but that list would be outdated before my head hit the pillow tonight. I'd rather give you tools and tips for finding your own sources, since those sources vary so greatly by state and situation. Finding a way to switch to meat and other products from humanely raised animals will involve working together with other people to create the social camaraderie of a bowling team instead of the isolation of the guy in the far lane, bowling alone. The tips presented here may slow your life down to the point you might actually tie on an apron and cook a meal or two in your own kitchen. And hopefully these tips will offer you a satisfying plunge into a pleasant pool of refreshing water, as opposed to our earlier submersion in sheep dip.

# Get Real about
# Your Goals

··· ··· ······ ··· ···

As a child I played "Captain, May I?" with my sister and the neighborhood kids. One kid would stand a set distance from the rest of us, then we'd each ask the captain's permission to take one big step forward, or perhaps two skips, or three hops, or maybe ten baby steps. The goal was to be the first to reach and tag the captain. You had to freeze between moves; if the captain caught you moving, you'd be sent back to the beginning. It was always the energetic kids who tried to reach the captain quickly with big leaps or clever steps who got sent back. The one who patiently requested and took only baby steps usually reached her goal first.

Taking baby steps, or setting small, realistically achievable goals, means you'll have a better chance of succeeding. Although I've gotten very good at paying attention and wasting less meat, my project to switch from factory meat to happy meat has had mixed results. My initial goal to entirely replace factory meat with happy meat, although noble and compassionate, was naïve. I tried taking a big leap instead of baby steps.

The Japanese have a strategy for change that relies on making small, continuous improvements—*kaisan.* When humans make a change, even if it's a positive one, we activate fear in our emotional brain (which apparently is different from our thinking brain). If this fear is great enough, our fight-or-flight instinct kicks in, and most of us will run from that change like sheep running from a wolf. No wonder I'd so often failed to lose weight. With my fear of "I'll never be able to do this," I obviously triggered the flight response, and off I went to the box of Fudgesicles. But if I take tiny steps, as advocated by *kaisan,* I'm less likely to set off that urge to flee, so my thinking brain remains in charge and I move forward.

·When it comes to meat, biting off more than you can chew (sorry!) and activating that fight-or-flight instinct means you'll end up right back where you started—eating only factory meat. Each of us must take stock of our own lives and the resources available to us, and then from there we must craft goals that make sense. I'm lucky enough to live in the country, where I'm surrounded by farmers, so buying meat directly from other farmers is easy. Our friends Lori and Al raise delicious chickens with care and consideration and butcher the animals right on their farm, reducing the stresses animals experience from transportation: Robin used to raise hogs conventionally, but without antibiotics and growth hormones. She's gotten out of the business, so I'm on the prowl for another source for pork.

We buy beef from Drew, who raises cattle fairly conventionally because he doesn't have enough land on which to graze them. He gives them access to a small pasture when he can, then feeds them a mixture of grain and hay. But the animals aren't given drugs and are treated with respect, and that's enough for me. My available resources, therefore, include farmers. I love these guys and am so proud to be one of them.

It's the convenience food that trips me up. To eat at a restaurant that serves humanely raised meat, I must drive thirty miles. The nearest vegetarian restaurant is sixty-five miles away. From a gas consumption point of view, this doesn't make much sense to me. I also don't have time to drive sixty-five miles for a meal. The Schwan's guy, however, drives right up to my front door in his pale yellow freezer truck loaded with convenience food made from factory meat and hands me a catalog. I point to the glossy photos of beef tamales, crispy chicken strips, and turkey medallions, and two minutes later those items are in my freezer. Is convenience going to trump compassion every time?

No, but in my life, with my cooking interests and skills, I now see that the real will never entirely match the ideal, since convenience food will always make up at least some part of my diet. Here's where treating *ourselves* with compassion becomes important. Just because the real doesn't always match the ideal is no reason to beat ourselves up and quit, or worse yet, not even try. When making art or music, sometimes the images or notes in our heads don't always make it onto the paper or into the instrument just the way we imagined it. The reality of raising kids might differ from what you expect. Relationships, even good ones, often fall short of our ideal relationship. The same is true of changing the way you eat meat. If your real doesn't entirely live up to your ideal, it's not the end of the world. At least we're all moving forward toward our goal of improving the lives of animals and reducing our environmental hoofprint.

Before you set your baby-step goals, take a personal inventory of your thoughts about eating meat. Make a list of everything you've learned about how livestock animals live, how they die, and do this by specific animal. What bothers you the most? Is it that sows are kept in cages or that chicken slaughter is so inhumane? This is how sick our modern food system has become, that

caring people who've opened their eyes must choose between torturing an animal during its life or possibly torturing it during its
death. Heck of a choice.

Avoid setting absolutes in what you will or will not accept in
your happy meat. Setting absolutes, when it comes to food, can
backfire. New York City banned trans fat from restaurants, wanting to reduce the health risks from artificially created fats. But
trans fat also occurs naturally in butter, meat, milk, and cheese,
and in fact, many researchers believe these natural trans fats are
healthy. Yet to meet the NYC requirements, bakers and restaurants have to remove natural fats like butter and replace it with
processed fats like palm oil and margarine. A representative from
the National Dairy Council said, "Things like a NY ban on trans
fat create hysteria, and when you create hysteria people overreact,
and when people overreact they start taking whole food groups
out of their diet because there might be a little trans fat in it."[1]

Compassionate carnivores need to fight the same hysteria surrounding meat—No grain! No feedlots! No antibiotics! If you eat
any meat at all raised in the factory system, you are eating meat
that has been given a steady dose of antibiotics and finished
on grain in a feedlot. So while you may not like every practice
a small farmer uses, most are surely improvements over the factory system.

To suddenly expect all non-factory farms to conform to some
perfect standard could put you in the New York City trans fat situation, where you are rejecting something that is better than what
you currently eat. If you believe organic meat is the only way to
go, and you can find a local source, excellent. But if you can't,
should you really be eating organic meat transported from a thousand miles away, or should you be eating meat from a sustainable
farmer sixty miles away, and encourage that farmer to eventually
go organic? As a compassionate carnivore, any move you make
*away* from factory meat is a huge step in the right direction.

I've drawn the line at pork. Unless I consume it by accident as a hidden ingredient, or find myself in a social situation where the host will be upset if I decline, I prefer not to eat pork unless I know where it came from. That image of the white sow at the state fair has never left me. I am not an absolutist, however, for you'll find a jar of real bacon bits in my fridge door. I try to fry up turkey bacon for our spinach salads, but some days I just don't have the time. Everyone draws a different line. One friend sets as her guideline "Four feet, no eat." Another seeks out animals that cannot, as yet, be raised in factories, like bison or elk.

I find self-help books one of the most irritating genres on the planet. I cannot stand their claims of "Get rich in five minutes!" or "Lose weight by eating ten pounds of chocolate a day!" or "Become the Best Lover in the World in Five Easy Moves!"

What's even more irritating than the books themselves is my compulsion to read them. Though I stay away from the ones whose covers promise diet and romantic and financial success, I am totally drawn in by the ones touting self-improvement. They always have great advice about setting goals, and it always includes the tip to set specific goals, not vague ones.

The statement "I want to eat more humanely raised meat" is so vague, you won't know what to do next. Try something more specific, like "I want to eat one meal a month from animals raised humanely." Or "I will buy three dozen eggs a month that come from uncaged hens." Or "I will make four phone calls this month in search of happy meat." Or "I will find a source for pasture-raised butter."

You can't really measure your success if your goal is to "eat more humanely raised meat." But if your goal is to home-cook two meals a month from humanely raised meat, you can measure this. Of course, once you've met your goal, don't stop there. Continue challenging yourself to replace more and more meat from animals raised in factories with meat from animals raised humanely.

Whether you invoke "Captain, May I?" or *kaisan,* set reasonable goals as you begin. Remember that sustainable applies not only to a farming method, but also to creating something that lasts, that continues. Creating lasting sustainable change is more important than creating temporary dramatic change.

# Don't Bowl
# Alone

••• ••• •••••• ••• •••

IN THE DISTANT past, humans used to understand that when it came to finding food, it was better to do it together, an instinct we've since lost. Two million years ago our hominoid ancestors began eating meat. Since we hadn't yet figured the whole hunting thing out, our source of meat was carcasses we stole from other carnivores, a fairly creepy practice known as kleptoparasitism. As scientist Blaire Van Valkenburgh writes, "The ability to throw rocks with force and accuracy would have been a major innovation and might have allowed groups of *Homo* to become kleptoparasites, actually driving smaller groups of large predators from their kills, as lions, hyenas and wild dogs do today."[2]

Once our group of fierce hominoids frightened away another predator and claimed its meat, they learned to work together to pull it apart. Since man lacked the kind of teeth needed to break up the carcass, as well as the tools to do so, they each grabbed a leg and yanked. They probably also watched each other's back so a saber-toothed cat or lion or pack of hyenas couldn't sneak up and make a meal out of *them*. Thank goodness we no longer have to climb up into a tree and steal some poor leopard's rotting gazelle carcass in order to eat meat. But, whereas throughout history, hunting down food was a group activity, today we do it basically by ourselves, and in supermarkets, not jungles.

Robert Putnam writes about how participation in group activities in this country has plummeted the last thirty years as more of us stay home with the TV and frozen pizza. His book *Bowling Alone* uses as its main metaphor the guy bowling alone, too busy or too disinterested to actually commit to joining a team and bowling with others.[3] Participation in sports, civic organizations, social organizations, and political organizations has dropped. We do more things alone now than ever before, including dealing with meat. Finding meat for our families is a solitary act—drive to the supermarket, grab a package from the meat section, and you're done.

Becoming a more compassionate carnivore will be easier if we remember those hominoids working together and find someone to share the experience with us. Not only for support, but for the more practical reason that if you want to buy a side of beef directly from a farmer, you likely won't have room for 250 pounds of meat in your Amana side-by-side.

Hunting down meat together can be a satisfying and connecting social experience. Our friend Amelia wanted to buy a quarter of a humanely raised beef steer but didn't need that much meat, so she got on the phone and found eight families willing to split it. The act of coming together to divide up the meat, then share recipes, then cook for each other brought those eight families together in a community, one that never would have existed if they'd just bought their beef at the grocery store.

Who might you look for? Like-minded people at work, in your office building, at church, parents of your kids' friends, neighbors, or even your children. Will your children be harmed by looking more closely at their meat, where it comes from and how it's raised? Cowboy poet and former veterinarian Baxter Black thinks not:

> Ninety-seven percent of our population eats meat. Yet most urban kids have no idea where it comes from. Modern society has separated the ham from the burger, the chicken from the nugget, and the hot fudge sundae from the holstein.
>
> We have sanitized our children's world. So they can eat without considering the sacrifice and service that domestic animals provide to humans' well-being. For those who might think urban people are not capable of dealing with the blunt truth of animal production, I suggest that they are. From the beginning of civilization until fifty years ago . . . people learned from childhood the intricate intimacy of raising and dealing with animals. . . . Country kids still maintain this close natural relationship. It instills respect and a sacred responsibility toward those animals in their care who are destined for the food chain.[4]

Then there's the hysterical *New Yorker* cartoon of a mother and child in the kitchen with a live cow draped over the center island, looking a bit weary of the whole thing. The mom says to the kid, "Mommy wants you to know where your food comes from."

According to Putnam, when people begin making connections with one another, establishing bonds of trust and understanding and building community, they are creating social capital. This is just a fancy phrase for networks of relationships that weave individuals into communities. Social capital can be bonding capital, sort of like Super Glue that brings people already part of a community closer together—birds of a feather stick together.

Then there's bridging capital, which is more difficult to form, but it unites more diverse groups, bridging splits in our communities. So with the simple act of finding a friend to share a side of beef with, you're building bonding capital. If you usually only hang out with Democrats but find yourself connecting with the Republican in the next cubicle over because you're both interested in undermining factory farms, you're building bridging capital.[5]

In a country where it's hard to talk to strangers, simply introduce a dog into the equation and two strangers can talk to each other. Our love of animals helps us bridge deep political and social divides, and I believe this can be true whether that animal is a pet to be kissed repeatedly or an animal raised on a farm and destined to be eaten.

Another way to avoid bowling alone is to move onto a ranch with twenty-six other families. Maytag Mountain Ranch, a three-thousand-acre working cattle ranch in Hillside, Colorado, is selling twenty-seven house lots. The residents will be able to participate in as much of the ranch work as they want, from herding the cattle to feeding the chickens. Each resident will receive a quarter steer every year, and lots of fresh eggs. Of course, the real estate price tag is incredibly steep, but it's an intriguing concept and will ensure you a supply of pasture-raised meat.[6]

I have this dream that instead of land at the fringes of cities being developed into one-acre lots with McMansions, the developers would keep the lots smaller and circle them around a large common grazing area. The new neighborhood could raise its own beef, pork, and chicken; kids would learn respect for meat animals by caring for them; and residents could relax because they'd know what's gone into their meat.

Your options are limited only by your time and imagination. I know it's American to go it alone, to be independent, but when it comes to becoming a more compassionate carnivore, you'll need help. Imagine exchanging recipes. Imagine piling the kids into the neighbor's van and spending Saturday visiting a farm. Imagine having a farmer come to your church group and showing a PowerPoint presentation of her farm.

There's nothing wrong with doing this alone. But when it comes to bowling, who's having more fun—the guy in the lane by himself, or the team of four guys wearing loud shirts and laughing up a storm?

The same can be true for eating meat. You could go it alone and be fine, or you could gather a team around you and learn together.

# Start Where You Live

··· ··· ······ ··· ···

THE EASIEST WAY to seek out more humanely raised meat is to start in your own backyard (and as we'll see, some people take that very literally). Are there any grocery stores nearby that are advertising humanely or locally raised meat? You can find out more about where the meat comes from by simply calling and asking, and then giving it a try. If you buy, the stores will continue to supply it. If your local stores don't carry it, start requesting that they do.

While most farmers markets tend to focus on fruits and vegetables, more of them are also featuring meat, but there may not be enough to meet demand. A farmer cannot just show up and begin selling meat out of the back of a truck like she can vegetables or fruit. Meat spoils if it's not handled properly, and spoiled meat makes people sick. To sell meat, a farmer must apply for a meat handler's license. The requirements for this license may vary by state, but to qualify, farmers must buy the equipment necessary to pick up the meat, store it, and transport it safely to the market. This means commercial freezers, an enclosed trailer lined with a washable surface, and a generator to power the freezers. Perhaps this is why many small farmers have hesitated to jump into the farmers market scene. Others just aren't cut out for talking with strangers all day long every weekend. To find out if there are farmers markets in your community, use the USDA's Web site: http://ams.usda.gov/farmersmarkets/map.htm.

A few restaurants have begun paying attention. The Chipotle chain advertises that it serves only humanely raised meat. Wolfgang Puck has decided to make the same switch. Many chefs, in fact, are buying and raising their own herds of cattle to ensure the cuts and flavor of the meat they want for their restaurants. Chefs Mario Batali and Adam Perry Lang have created a company to produce humanely raised animals that are "pampered from the farm to the slaughterhouse."[7] These are just a few examples of restaurant professionals who are making commitments to better quality of life for the animals that feed us.

Portland, Oregon, is a great example of what can happen when restaurateurs, customers, and farmers establish relationships with one another. During the last fifteen years a number of innovative chefs have moved to Portland and begun cooking using local ingredients in season. And what kind of farmers are they working with? As reported in the *New York Times,* "Many of the older farmers came from the Bay Area in the 1970s with a vision of sustainable agriculture, and they have continued to adhere to those principles."[8] Shifting from factory-raised meat to humanely raised hasn't hurt the economy of Portland restaurants one bit.

Chefs are leading the way in eating as much of an animal as possible, calling it the "whole-animal diet." Writer Tom Philpott explains in *Gastronomica:* "If we must do the dirty deed of raising an animal to kill it, then we owe it to the animal to wring as much gustatory joy as possible out of the process."[9]

Cooking all parts of the carcass has become a badge of honor among chefs, and although this might strike some carnivores as taking the whole idea of not wasting anything a bit *too* far, others may find it exotic. Chefs—professional and home—cook up beef kidneys, heart, tongue, and stomach (tripe). They find ways to prepare the head, tail, feet, entrails, and internal organs. The magazine *Plenty* calls this "nose to tail eating." Chef Anthony Bourdain refers to cooking "the nasty bits." According to *Plenty*, "Critics coo over celebrity chef Mario Batali's tripe, beef cheeks, and lamb tongue; forums about offal abound on foodie websites."[10] Chef Chris Cosentino shares his experiences through his blog at http://offalgood.com. It's a great place to go if you need a recipe for cooking duck testicles.

Chefs have also discovered unlaid eggs. Stay with me here. When laying hens' production slows way down, thanks to age, they are butchered and processed into chicken soup. A New York chef, Dan Barber, discovered that some of the butchered hens contained eggs about to be laid. Some were as small as a marble, others the size of a regular egg but with the shell not yet formed. Calling them "immature" eggs, Barber prepares them for his restaurants, describing their taste as "deep, concentrated flavor, a hint of sweetness, but not overly rich."[11]

Once you've investigated area restaurants, your next step is to look for a CSA, which stands for community-supported agriculture. This is like subscribing to a farm. While most CSAs sell vegetables and fruit, more are adding meat. You pay a membership fee, which the cash-desperate farmer uses to plant crops and pay labor at the season's beginning. In return, you receive a share of the farm's harvest. The CSA nearest us shows up once a week at a local park, and the members stop by to retrieve that week's share of veggies.

Meat can be handled the same way. If I were to run a CSA for meat, I'd collect membership fees, using the money to feed and care for the animals, and to pay the processor to slaughter the animal and package the meat. Members would then receive a certain number of pounds. Visit www.localharvest.org to find the CSAs near you.

When it comes to eggs, some enterprising city dwellers are raising laying hens in their backyards. In 1910, 43 percent of all

households raised their own chickens and eggs.[12] Today hardly anyone does, even those people living out in the country. But some
cities, like Seattle, Portland, Minneapolis, and Madison, Wisconsin,
are changing their animal ordinances in response to the growing
movement of raising hens for eggs. A group of Madison folks, Mad
City Chickens (http://madcitychickens.com) are not only interested
in eating better eggs, but they're creative as well. Every summer they
hold an annual chicken coop tour, where Madison residents, armed
with maps, can visit urban chicken coops.[13] The one I saw was designed to look like a saloon, complete with swinging doors and a
hitching post out front. Although the hens are in an enclosure, they
have plenty of room and do not seem caged. When the weather is
nice, their owners let them roam the backyard, as long as there aren't
any hawks hanging around in the tree branches.

The magazine *Backyard Poultry* provides tips and information
for raising chickens. A woman in West Oakland, California,
helps low-income families raise chickens as a source of healthy
food. A bakery owner in Berkeley started raising chickens in his
backyard to feed them breadcrumbs from the bakery. Most raise
the chickens for eggs, but when hens become unproductive,
some backyard poultry practitioners butcher them for meat.
The older the chicken and the more exercise it's had in its life, the
more flavor and texture in the meat.[14]

The key to this urban poultry movement is that it's all local—
you can't get much more local than your own backyard—and
that people are working together, sharing what they know about
coop construction and design, chicken feed requirements, and
chicken health. They aren't bowling alone.

The humanely raised or organic meat you find may have come
from across the ocean. It's up to you whether that's okay just in
the short run, or if it's okay with you in the long run. If you don't
like the idea of eating meat that has so many transportation miles
on it, then your next option is to find your own farmer.

# Finding a
# Farmer

··· ··· ······ ··· ···

MOST OF YOU likely won't know a small farmer. Perhaps your neighbor or a work colleague has a cousin once removed on her mother's side who knows a farmer. But that's not very likely, either, given that less than 1 percent of the population farms. Also, while sustainable farming is catching on, there still aren't that many of us. *Time* estimated that between 2001 and 2006 more than one thousand U.S. ranchers switched their herds to an all-grass diet, but pasture-raised beef still represents less than 1 percent of beef sold in the country.[15]

Although more farmers are starting meat CSAs across the country, or beginning to participate in farmers markets, you don't need to wait for a farmer to find you. Instead, get together a group of people who are willing to purchase a set quantity of beef, pork, chicken, or lamb, then find a farmer who is willing to raise the animals for you. People form buying clubs to purchase staples like flour and sugar and pasta in bulk, so why not do the same for meat?

Whether you're looking for a CSA or an individual farmer, don't focus solely on online resources, since according to a report

212 The Compassionate Carnivore

I heard on National Public Radio the other day, only 55 percent of farmers have access to the Internet. If farmers are selling their meat as a commodity, they have no need for direct contact with consumers. Other farms are too small to advertise, so they rely on word of mouth. (That would be Melissa and me.)

Where do you find small farmers? Here are a few places to try:

- Sustainable agriculture departments or associations. These were started to provide support for sustainable farmers. While many have begun connecting consumers with farmers, not all are yet set up to do so. Be patient, since these organizations are not for your benefit, but for the farmers. See the list of Organizations and Web Sites for Finding Farmers in the Resources section.
- Web sites focusing on sustainable, humanely raised or organic meat. You'll find some in the same section.
- Ask other farmers at farmers markets if they know anyone else who might be raising livestock humanely, but who don't presently sell their meat at a farmers market.

As more carnivores wake up and start looking for non-factory meat, dairy, and eggs, things are going to get tight. It might be frustrating tracking down a farmer only to find she has nothing to sell you, since some farmers won't be licensed to do this, others won't be interested in selling directly to consumers, and others will have run out of product.

This has already happened with cage-free eggs now that Whole Foods, Burger King, and Ben & Jerry's want to sell or use only cage-free eggs. It's going to take awhile for supply to catch up with demand. Egg producers will not be getting any encouragement from the United Egg Producers, whose president said, "There is a lot of talk about cage-free, but are people actually buying them? I think the consumer walking into the grocery store sees cage-free and they cost two or three times more and they don't buy them."[16]

According to this organization, a few years ago about 2 percent of the 279 million laying hens in this country were cage-free; now we're up to about 5 percent. It's been estimated to cost about eight dollars per bird to build a conventional cage operation, and about thirty dollars per bird to build a cage-free operation.[17]

Will meat from animals raised sustainably, out on a pasture, cost more? Probably, but becoming a more conscientious carnivore is about building relationships, not about finding the cheapest steak raised on grass. It takes more labor to raise animals on pasture, more thinking, more consideration, more running around chasing after animals that have broken the rules. Instead of shipping an animal that's sick, a sustainable farmer is more likely to spend the time and money to cure it.

Small farmers aren't large enough to realize the economies of scale the big guys do. Also, small farmers don't receive the government subsidies that large farmers receive. The largest 8 percent of farms, those making more than $250,000 per year, receive nearly 50 percent of the government subsidy payments.[18] Add in those farmers making more than $100,000, and you have 17 percent of farmers receiving nearly 75 percent of all payments. Meat from small farms costs more because we're paying for the externalities, and our profit must come entirely from our products, not from government subsidies.

Here's conservative author Rod Dreher's take on the idea of paying more: "Does it cost more? Sure. But we want to be able to trust that the meat is clean, and we feel good about paying a little more to avoid being complicit in the factory-farming system that ruins landscapes and traditional farming communities. Cheap chicken is not worth a compromised conscience."[19]

Joel Salatin, a successful sustainable farmer and marketer in Virginia, points out why people shouldn't balk at paying more for their food: "We wouldn't for a minute, say, 'Let's go to the cheapest church in town; let's hire the cheapest preacher we can get.' We wouldn't say, 'Let's go to the cheapest brain surgeon.' But we're very happy to put on the lowest respect level and honor level the stewards of our food system and the stewards of our landscape."[20]

It costs money to either change a farm's production system or increase its output. Before making this investment, most farmers will worry, Is this just a fad? Will I expand my operation only to find people have moved on and no longer care about grass-fed, or humanely raised, or cage-free? And while growth will be necessary to meet the increasing demand, getting too big will be a risk for every farm.

If farmers do make the commitment to grow, they can't increase their supply overnight, so be patient. If a publisher runs out of a book, it can print more. If a clothing store runs out of jeans, the manager orders more and they appear. But when a farmer runs out of meat, it takes a little longer to refill the freezer. First, the animals must breed or be artificially inseminated. Then it takes twenty-one days to "make" a baby chick, three and a half months for a piglet, five months for a lamb, and around nine months for a calf.

The farmer must then raise the animals, which will take six to eight weeks for a chicken, four months for a hog, nine months for a lamb, and from eighteen to twenty-four months for a beef steer, depending on what it's fed. So if the entire country suddenly decides meat from animals raised humanely is the way to go, please don't get your shorts in a bundle because we've all run out of meat. Remember that farmers raise only what they think they can sell. We usually finish half of our lambs and sell the rest to other farmers to finish. But if we see an increasing demand for our lamb, we'll finish all of them. Basically, if you let small farmers know you're out there, interested in buying our meat, we'll make more.

A quick word about farmers: we are not a homogeneous bunch. There are large farmers who treat their animals with kindness and respect; there are small farmers who abuse animals. Some farmers are willing to do what's necessary to care properly for the environment, while there are others who learned as children to dump their old appliances in the gully behind the house, and that's what they'll continue to do. Many large farmers don't like the corporate farm system, but either don't know how to change or don't have the financial freedom to do so. Many small farmers just keep doing things the way their parents did them, continuing the conventional model without question.

There are farmers with five million dollars' worth of equipment on their place—tractors, combines, haying equipment, trucks, and skid loaders—while the neighbor down the road might have nothing more than a team of golden Percherons tossing creamy manes as they pull a plow. Some farmers chose this profession because they love it; others inherited the job and land from their parents and hate it.

Farmers aren't perfect and don't wear halos. Just because a person farms doesn't mean he or she is going to share my philosophy on animals or the environment or on eating meat. Farmers are fiercely independent and hate being told what to do.

An industry representative came to our sheep producers' meeting one January and bemoaned the wide range of breeds, shapes, sizes, and meat quality of the sheep we all raised. "If only the sheep people would all raise the same breed of sheep," the man said, "like the beef guys raise Angus or dairy guys raise Holstein, then life would be so much easier for the processors and agribusiness people." He wanted us all to agree to raise just Dorsets or just Columbias or just Targhee sheep.

We looked around the room at one another. At the next table sat Dan, who raised pony-sized, black-faced Suffolks to show at county fairs. Those fussy things wouldn't last a day out on pasture, so *no way,* I thought. No meat customer's going to pay me for all that air under a tall Suffolk. Dan probably looked at us thinking, "Those two women raise those shrimpy commercial sheep with short legs and white faces; what a waste of time."

In the space of about two seconds, every shepherd in the room considered every other breed raised by others in the room and quickly decided they weren't changing a thing, damn it.

Farmers are like that.

Successful farmers can perform lots of jobs. A farmer must be a vet, animal specialist, crop expert, nutritionist, mechanic, electrician, truck driver, commodity trader, accountant, marketing and promotion expert, safety engineer, employer, manager, and creative thinker.

Not surprisingly, not all of these hats fit well on every farmer's head. Some call the vet at the first sign of illness or birth problems, having no intention of ever sticking an arm into a cow's backside and delivering a calf. That would be me. Some farmers don't know everything about engines and must rely on patient neighbors or the tractor repair guy who makes farm calls. Jeff, thank you.

Not only will you have to look hard for farmers and be patient once you find them, but farmers, if they are going to get on the sustainable bandwagon, will have to invest in their farms, and possibly change how they operate. Build relationships with farmers. Give them a little leeway if their places aren't perfect, or if their marketing materials are photocopies instead of four-color print jobs. Get on their mailing lists. Offer to help produce the farm's newsletter or get an e-letter started. Tell us what you want, then give us time to grow your meat. Put down a healthy deposit on future meat deliveries so the small farmer has some cash to work with. Farmers can't afford to change or grow if customers say they're interested but then disappear. Since we're in this for the long haul, let us know you are, too.

Not to put undue pressure on you, but you don't have lots of time. Many small farmers are disappearing because they can't thrive in a food system designed now for the big guys. So don't wait until your kids are out of college, or until you retire and have loads of free time. The only small farms left by then may just be hobby farms.

While motoring up the St. Johns River north of Jacksonville, Florida, in my brother-in-law's sailboat, we passed a huge, ocean-going ship that had been loaded and now needed help turning around so it could head back out to sea. Three little tugboats, industriously churning up the water behind them, were slowly turning that ship around.

You're the tugboat. You may be just one person out of 300 million, but you have the power to churn things up and turn at least some farmers in the direction you need them to go.

# Visiting
# a Farm

··· ··· ······ ··· ···

SO YOU'VE MADE the phone calls, sent off the e-mails, and read the state lists of sustainable farmers. However you did it, you've found a farmer you can connect with. You like how she raises her animals, she's not that far away, and you're ready to go check the place out.

Visiting a farm can be an amazing experience. You will see actual farm animals. You may see actual farm animals performing sexual congress. You may see hens pecking the ground. You may see bins of grain, stacks of hay, or acres of pasture. You may see broken equipment, piles of unrecognizable material, perhaps a compost pile, a manure pile waiting to be spread. There will be equipment standing around waiting to be moved or fixed or sold or towed away. There will be scrap metal and scrap wood and extra twine and empty buckets and broken fence posts and lots of tools.

If it's been a bad day, you might even see a dead animal. Farmers have no control over an animal's sudden death. Try not to shriek or cry, making the farmer feel worse than she already does.

I've been on farms where the dog drags up some unidentifiable body part from some unidentifiable animal. Be cool. Act like you see this sort of thing all the time.

Keep in mind that farms won't be spotless. I remember touring farms before we started ours, and thinking how scandalous it was that the barn rafters were always thick with unsightly cobwebs. I resolved that when we had a barn, I would keep those rafters free of cobwebs.

You should see our barn. Our cobwebs have cobwebs. They are so coated in dirt, they've taken on an almost lacy appearance. Some might even be considered modern art.

As you tour a farm, don't wrinkle up your nose at the dust in the barn, the cobwebs, the chicken poop on the feed bin. As long as none of these things are anywhere near where your meat might be stored, relax.

Here are a few more tips to make sure your farm visit goes smoothly.

1. *Call first.* We might be napping. In fact, if it's right after lunch, I guarantee we'll be napping. There's something about working outside in the sun and wind and cold for hours that can zap you; twenty minutes is a great little recharge.
2. *Show up when you say you will.* Farmers are busy, so it's really frustrating to hang around the house waiting for you when they could be using that time doing something out on pasture. At least call if you're delayed. Bring cookies as a peace offering for your tardiness. In fact, bring cookies even if you're on time.
3. *Leave your pets at home.* Yes, I know Buster would love to run and stretch his citified legs, but letting him chase chickens and snap them up and shake them until they're dead will not win you the Good Visitor Award. If the dog's in the car, leave him there. Don't even ask.

We learned this lesson when we held a one-year-birthday party for our border collie, inviting two other border collies to the party. One jumped the fence and chased the pregnant sheep. The other jumped the fence and chased the pregnant goats.

4. *Wear the ugly boots.* Even if you've never stepped on another farm your entire life, a farmer may ask you to slip a pair of clear plastic boots over your shoes. Disease can spread easily from farm to farm and devastate a flock or herd, so hush up and learn to shuffle-walk so the boots stay on.

5. *Bring well-behaved children.* If you tell your children to stop chasing the chickens, please notice if they have actually stopped. If you don't control your children, then the farmer must, and it tarnishes our carefully cultivated image as nice people.

6. *Wear appropriate clothing.* Don't appear in sandals or flip-flops or, god forbid, *barefoot,* and expect your walk through a chicken's/duck's/sheep's world to be a pleasant and pristine experience. Of course, if you like the feel of duck poop squishing through your toes, who am I to judge?

7. *Bring cookies.* Oops, I repeat myself.

8. *Pay attention to gates.* If you go through a gate that's open when you get there, leave it open. If you go through a gate that's closed when you get there, please close it behind you. If you're at the tail end of a group of people and don't know if the gate was open or closed, ask.

9. *Don't argue with the farmer.* If the farmer casually mentions that her chickens have recently begun flying up into the chicken house rafters and crapping on her head, don't tell the farmer you've seen *Chicken Run* ten times and know perfectly well that chickens can't fly. She will lead you into the chicken house, where you will gaze at the chickens up in the rafters, and they will crap on your head.

10. *Ask questions.* Most farmers love to talk about their animals and their operations. If they didn't, you likely wouldn't be visiting that farm in the first place. The more people who understand farming, the better the chances it will survive both as a lifestyle and as a business. Farmers are used to answering lots of questions, even questions you might think are dumb. Don't be embarrassed to ask why that rooster suddenly jumped onto the back of that white hen. It's good to be curious.

When you ask questions, keep an open mind. You might learn something new about the animals. Just because a farming practice isn't sanctioned by a certifying body, or hasn't been mentioned in this book, or hasn't been written about in the *New York Times* doesn't mean it's bad or wrong. Remember that farmers are fiercely independent, and most of us have very good reasons for doing what we do on our farms. This is a business, and we've each figured out the best way to do business on the piece of land we own. What I do on the rolling hills of southeastern Minnesota may make no sense for a piece of land in western Montana or central Florida. If a particular practice makes you uncomfortable, ask for more information.

11. *Don't ask if this is a hobby farm.* Never assume a small farm is a hobby farm. I know I've said this before, but I'll say it again: Anyone who would work this hard on a hobby is insane.

12. *Show your gratitude for the visit.* Two tickets for an Alaskan cruise would be good. Or maybe new tires for the Farmall 706 tractor. Or if none of these are within your reach, cookies would be nice.

# Learning
# the Lingo

... ... ...... ... ...


FINDING A FARMER is much harder than actually communicating with one. All you need are a few basic questions to get the conversation started, and you're good to go. Farmers watch the same TV shows you do, read the same magazines, follow the same sports teams, vote, and most are highly educated. Despite the dictionary's alternate definition of *farmer* as "yokel or bumpkin," chances are pretty good you won't have to talk slowly or spell out the big words. So relax and have fun. What follows are some questions to ask farmers.

1. *How do you sell your meat?*
   Farmers can sell wholesale to you. This means she is selling you a live animal and taking it to the processor for you; then when the meat is ready, you pick it up. Federal regulations are strict about whether a farmer can actually bring the meat home and store it on the farm. That's why you may be expected to pick it up yourself—because the farmer might not be able to legally bring it home. In Minnesota we can now bring the meat home and sell it off the

farm without a meat handler's license, but every state will be different.

When a farmer sells wholesale, she is usually constrained by regulations to only sell whole or half animals rather than individual cuts like steaks or ground beef. As I've mentioned earlier, a whole hog would be 165 pounds of meat and a steer may be about 550 pounds of meat. A whole lamb would be about 40 pounds of meat. Because a steer is so large, farmers are allowed to sell quarters. You pay the farmer for the meat, and you pay the butcher to process the animal.

The next option for some farms is retail. The farmer will have a freezer on the farm and will be happy to sell you individual cuts. She'll charge more for the individual cuts because she's had to pay the processing charges, and because certain cuts are more desirable, so they can bring higher prices. Some farmers will put together convenience packs, where they choose the mix of cuts and then charge you less. Why? Because every part of an animal needs to be consumed, since it's wasteful to butcher an animal just for its T-bone steaks. I'll leave the exotic stuff to the chefs, but it's not a bad idea to try different, perfectly edible cuts. Since that animal has been killed to feed us, it seems the least we can do.

Which would you prefer—to buy individual cuts or a whole animal? It'd be great if you could start with a few cuts to make sure you like the taste, but not every farmer will be able to do this. However, if you are buying a whole hog with a group of people, you'll each have a small amount, which will help you decide if you want to buy more.

2. *How do you price your meat?*
Let's start with the method you're most familiar with—individual cuts on a per pound basis. You're used to buying ground beef for two dollars per pound or five dollars per

pound, or lamb chops for twelve dollars per pound. If a farmer can sell individual cuts, he'll price this way.

If you are buying wholesale, there likely will be two ways the farmer might charge you. One is by live weight. If the lamb weighs 130 pounds when it arrives at the butcher, you'll be charged a rate times 130. Another method is to charge by hanging weight. Once everything nonedible has been removed—head, hooves, insides, hide—the processor will weigh the carcass and charge you by the hanging weight.

3. *Do I pick up my meat at your farm, or do you deliver?*
   Doesn't hurt to ask, right? Expect to pay more for delivered meat.

4. *Are there any retail outlets where I can buy your meat?*
   Don't be surprised if the answer to this is no. Be patient. We're working on it.

5. *Where was the animal born? How did it come to be on your farm?*
   Some farmers raise animals from birth; others buy animals and finish them. Either is fine; the question just gives you more information about that farmer's operation.

6. *Please describe the animal's living conditions. Did it have access to pasture? How much of the time?*
   Though I'd like my meat to come from animals that have spent their entire lives on pasture, it's not a deal breaker as long as the animal has been cared for with compassion and hasn't been pumped full of growth hormones, antibiotics, and grain.

7. *What did the animal eat? All grass? All grain? A mix? If the animal ate grain, what percentage of the animal's diet was grain?*
   If an entirely grass-fed animal is important to you, then stick by your guns and keep looking until you find it.

8. *Where will the animal be processed?*
   The farmer may be lucky enough to have a processing plant thirty minutes away, or he may have to truck the animals

several hours. If this is the case, keep in mind that this factor is outside the farmer's control.

9. *Do you use antibiotics or growth hormones on a regular basis?*
   We use antibiotics to save an animal's life, but we then make sure that animal doesn't become part of our meat supply.

10. *Do you have an annual open house or visiting day?*
    Most small farmers have off-farm jobs, so they don't have a lot of free time to spend showing potential customers around the farm. This is why holding one day of open house might make more sense for them. If the farmer doesn't have an open house, ask the next question:

11. *Would you be willing to spend thirty minutes showing us your operation? I'm interested in buying from you, but would like to visit first.*
    Offer to pay him twenty dollars for his time.

This is just a possible list. You'll have other questions based on your own motivations for making the switch to meat raised by small farmers.

If you are buying wholesale, your next step is to talk to the butcher. Because you are getting the entire animal, or a share of it, you decide how you want the meat cut. This was such an intimidating step for me that when we began selling lamb, we worked out two basic packages with the processor so that our customers didn't have to make lots of individual decisions.

But most farmers will just give you the name of the processor and ask you to call and give them "the information." When we bought our first beef quarter from a friend, that's exactly what he did. So I called the processor and someone growled, "Hansen's Meat."

"Hi, my name is Catherine Friend, and I'm buying a quarter of the steer John Smith is bringing in on October first."

"What's your name?"

"Catherine Friend."

"Whose steer?"

"John Smith."

"When's that coming in?"

At this point I jam on my Patience Hat, which isn't a good fit for me. "October first."

"Okay, got it." Now I realize the guy has been scrawling all this information down as we spoke. Then he stuns me with, "So, whaddya want?"

I swallow. "I want a quarter of the steer John Smith is bringing in on October first." I hate not knowing what I am doing.

"Yeah, I got that. I mean how do you want it cut?"

"With a knife" pops into my head, but I wisely bite my tongue. Silence hums along the phone line, until finally I can't take it. "Look, I've never done this before. I have no idea what you need from me. I'd appreciate it if you could lead me through this."

"Oh yeah, no problem." Then he began a rapid-fire series of questions that I somehow answered, then gratefully hung up.

The guy was so used to dealing with people who'd been buying meat this way for years that he'd forgotten there might be a few of us out there who don't have a clue. So here's a list of possible questions a meat processor might ask you:

- How thick would you like your steaks cut? One inch? One and a half?
- How many steaks or chops per package?
- What size roasts do you want? How many people will you be serving?
- Do you want stew meat?
- How lean would you like your ground beef?
- Want the ground beef made into patties?
- Want anything smoked or deboned?
- Would you like the organs (liver, heart, kidneys)?
- Want the tongue (for beef)?

Once you've given the processor your cutting instructions, then it's your turn. Ask them what the processing charge will be. The more special services you choose, like smoking or deboning, the higher your cost. Ask them when the meat will be available to pick up. They might give you a date, or they might say they'll call you.

Then all you do is wait patiently, patting yourself on the back for your persistence, cleverness, bravery, and wisdom in buying meat directly from a farmer.

# Slow Food
# vs. Go Food

··· ··· ······ ··· ···

MELISSA WEARS ONLY practical clothes. The pants must have lots of pockets, and they must be big pockets. The shirts and jackets must have lots of pockets, and they must be big pockets. Most women's clothing has woefully small pockets, eliciting curses from her when she can't even fit her pliers into a pocket. Her idea of dressing up is to wear jeans she hasn't patched. She considers a tan-and-brown-plaid shirt to be loud.

So imagine my surprise the day I walked into the kitchen and found Melissa wearing an apron—a green ruffly thing that tied behind her in a big bow. I began to laugh hysterically.

Melissa looked down at the apron. "What?" she asked.

I still couldn't speak, but just pointed to the apron.

"It was my grandmother's. And I'm making bread, which can be messy, so I need to wear an apron."

"You're making bread?" I reached for a chair, feeling faint.

"Very funny, ha ha. Yes, I'm making bread, and I'm wearing an apron."

The apron might be a perfect metaphor for the changing life of a compassionate carnivore, because—you may want to sit down for this news—you will have to cook more. That was the biggest shock of all for this carnivore, since I adore convenience food, not because it tastes good, but simply because it's convenient.

As I sought to make the switch from factory meat to happy meat, as I struggled to pay more attention so I wasn't cursing factory farming one minute then burying my face in a factory-raised pork-chop-on-a-stick the next, I smacked right into the wall of convenience.

Convenience is darned hard to give up. In 1969 grocery stores offered an average of seven thousand products. Today they tempt us with more than fifty thousand products, most of which have made our food preparation considerably more convenient.[21] Take frosting. People used to make it from scratch, but then companies started making boxes of dry frosting mix, and suddenly frosting a cake was possible for us non-bakers. But soon that box mix took too much time, so now we buy the frosting already mixed up in a plastic tub. All we need to do is spread it. If that's too much work, you can buy pre-frosted cakes in the frozen dessert section of your grocery store. Nobody doesn't like Sara Lee.

Americans now spend more than $1 trillion on food every year, and more than 90 percent of that is spent on processed food.[22] This is an astounding figure, and does much to explain our resistance to making changes in how we eat. We currently eat one-fourth of our meals in restaurants. If you assume we eat three meals a day, or twenty-one meals a week, one-fourth of that is a little more than five. So we are eating five meals out and sixteen meals in. Of the meals we eat at home, two-thirds are takeout or prepared food. So during a seven-day period, five meals are eaten out of the house, eleven meals at home are takeout or prepared foods, and only five meals are home-cooked.

Our reliance on convenience foods has fueled the growth in factory farms. How? Instead of the old-fashioned local system where the consumer used to buy a hunk of cheese from a local dairy and perhaps build her own pizza, we instead buy our pizzas from DiGiorno, Tombstone, and Red Baron. According to Sherri Brooks Vinton, coauthor of *Real Food Revival*, large food companies can only afford to deal with large growers and producers who can guarantee huge shipments of the same ingredient, so small farmers are cut out of the picture.[23] For example, it takes the milk from sixteen thousand cows to supply Red Baron with its *daily* requirement of cheese topping for its pizzas; if Red Baron had to collect this amount of cheese from a thousand small farms instead of a few large ones, they'd go broke. But if we all bought cheese from small, local dairies and made our own pizza— *voilà*—support for small farms.

The definition of cooking has changed. Cooking used to mean "made at home from scratch." Cooking involved ingredients . . . things you mix together. But as historian Maureen Greenwald found, by 1991 the definition of cooking had slackened enough to include scrambling eggs, preparing a salad, boiling pasta, and microwaving a vegetable.[24] Today cooking from scratch includes using prepared ingredients. For me, sticking a frozen pizza in the oven is cooking.

Fifty years ago advertisers began blurring the line defining "homemade" cooking in an attempt to assure women that buying their products—convenience food—didn't make them less responsible wives and mothers, since in the 1950s it was all about being a responsible wife and mother. Campbell's wanted women to serve their canned soup instead of making it from scratch. Chef Boyardee wanted women to serve their canned spaghetti products. Companies began throwing "home-baked taste" and "home-cooked meal" into their ads, hoping that just by using the word "home," consumers would feel comfortable replacing real home-cooked meals with the convenience meals. The ads showed smiling families being fed these convenience foods by a proud mother.[25]

It worked. Convenience foods have become such an integral part of our lives that it's hard to imagine life without them. Our meals, however, no longer look like those ads, with the entire family gathered around the table. According to chef Alice Waters, 57 percent of the children in the United States never regularly share meals with their families.[26] Convenience foods have made it easy and possible to eat on the run, and that's exactly what we do.

When I was a kid, family meals were a time when my parents and my sister and I told one another about our day. We learned table manners. We learned to listen while another person talked. We'd laugh so hard that sometimes my sister and I thought our guts would burst, so we'd spontaneously jump up from the table and run around the living room until we calmed down. I'd try to read a novel by hiding it on my lap, but my parents set a "No Reading at the Table" rule. When my irrepressible sister would start waving her arms around like some sort of exotic dancer, violating the airspace around my head, I complained loudly enough that my parents then set a "No Arm Dancing at the Table" rule.

Perhaps we need to get back in touch with Vinton's idea that "Meals are more than a way to fill your belly; they can be an oasis in a hectic schedule, a planned time, each day, to sit, chat, and reflect on the day."[27]

Slowing down our lives in order to sit down and share a meal is one step, but eating more slowly will also increase our enjoyment of the food. Eating psychologist Marc David recommends that we make sure we get enough vitamin P in our diet—P for pleasure. Our brains and digestive systems produce endorphins—natural chemicals that make us feel good—and "the simple act of eating raises our levels of endorphins." The more endorphins in our digestive system, the more blood and oxygen will head there, leading to increased digestion and greater calorie burning.

But if we eat food too quickly, or "without awareness or with a helping of guilt," our central nervous systems only register minimal pleasure, releasing fewer endorphins. As a result, we're "physiologically driven to eat more . . . compelled to hunt down the pleasure we never fully receive."[28] So instead of wolfing down that burger, slow down, reflect on what you're eating, and let vitamin P take over.

As part of our march toward convenience, canned goods became a normal part of the kitchen, to be followed swiftly by frozen goods. Swanson and Sons, a poultry processor in Omaha, decided to take advantage of the fact that many homes had begun buying those newfangled refrigerator-freezers. One of the "Sons" saw a new container used by Pan American Airlines to serve dinner on long flights—an aluminum tray with different compartments for the separate parts of the meal—and thought that might work as a container for a precooked meal. Frozen TV dinners were born, and in just a few short years Americans shifted from communal meals where the family members actually talked to one another, to meals where people stuffed their faces with dinners while sitting in front of the TV, those aluminum containers balanced on TV trays. My sister and I loved our once-a-week TV meals; eating in front of the TV was exciting for us.

Unfortunately, according to the book *Poplorica,* a history of fads and inventions that shaped America, "The TV dinner helped set an expectation of speed and ease that food cooked from fresh ingredients couldn't possibly match."[29] Suddenly, convenience food was cool and homemade food was not.

As a market researcher reported to *Food Engineering* in 2000: "For the WWII generation, the attitude can be summed up as, 'I'm glad I don't need to cook anymore.' For Baby Boomers it's been, 'I wish I had time to cook.' For Generation X, it's, 'What, me cook?' Generation Y wonders, 'What's cooking?'"[30]

Convenience does not come without a price. Remember those nasty externalities? If a meat source is very convenient for you, it was likely not very pleasant for the animal or the environment or the factory's neighbors. All three pay the price so that you can grab some takeout on your way home, or throw a frozen meal into the oven.

Economists love graphs that show the relationship between two events. If event A happening more often causes event B to happen less often, the two events are inversely related—one goes up, the other goes down. If event A rising causes event B to go up, they are directly related. An example of this would be as incomes rise, so do purchases of expensive cars. As income levels rise in developing countries, so do purchases of meat.

Convenience and the externalities of factory meat are directly related. As your convenience goes up, your consumption of factory meat goes up. The higher your factory meat consumption, the higher the amount of externalities created by modern agriculture that you're responsible for. If buying meat another way results in less convenience for you, the externalities associated with your meat consumption should decrease. You bypass the restaurant, which is highly convenient, and thaw a pound of hamburger you bought from a small farmer, which might have been a less convenient activity for you.

That's an economist's way of delivering bad news, by burying it in a graph, but there is just no getting around this fact: if a carnivore is going to switch from eating factory meat to eating meat from animals raised humanely, and you don't have a restaurant down the street available for all of your meals, you're going to have to cook more out of your freezer. Will cooking fit into your already busy schedule? Probably not. Something is going to have to give. You might have to slow down.

Lots of people are doing it. Founded in Italy in response to the growing spread of fast food, the Slow Food Movement supports the idea that we can use food for a "slower and more harmonious rhythm of life." The movement seeks to "catalyze a broad cultural shift away from the destructive effects of an industrial food system and fast life toward the regenerative cultural, social, ecological and economic benefits of a sustainable food system." This movement has now expanded into 45 countries, has 560 local branches, and more than 65,000 members. I love that the organization's members consider themselves not consumers, but coproducers, because "by being informed about how our food is produced and actively supporting those who produce it, we become a partner in the production process."[31]

No wonder this organization has grown so much. The idea of slowing down, of being partners with the farmers, isn't radical . . . it's returning us to where we should have been before factory farming took us off track. Would it really be so bad if you slowed your life down even a teensy bit? If you took charge of the ingredients of your food instead of letting corporations stuff you and your family, like baby birds, full of sugar, corn products, chemicals, and meat from really, really unhappy animals? If you shut off the TV for thirty minutes and have the family sit down around the table?

The most rewarding way to make the switch is to dig through your great-grandmother's trunk in the attic and find an apron. Or buy a new one with a funny saying on the front, or maybe a see-through apron—whatever it takes for you to put one on. Bravely enter your kitchen, with your children or spouse playing some supporting role. Put on that apron and start cooking again. My version of cooking is to grill meat, make a salad, or steam some veggies, and we're good to go. Julia Child I am not, but I received such an excellent Elvis apron for my birthday that it doesn't matter. Have apron, will cook.

I have not removed all prepackaged or precooked food from our lives, nor do I intend to. Today I have a tight schedule, so I'll be steaming some beef tamales sold to me by the nice man in the yellow Schwan's truck. But yesterday I made pesto chicken using Lori's chicken. Tomorrow it's hamburgers from Drew's beef. Tomorrow night it's boxed couscous with lemon juice and scallions. The day after that I'm thawing Robin's pork roast for my slow cooker.

Here's where that freezer comes in handy. If you have plenty of humanely raised meat on hand, you'll be more successful meeting your goals. The meat in my freezer won't cook itself, however, so I must give thought to the week ahead. I thaw meat the day before I need it. I'm getting more creative with ingredients. I sometimes try new recipes, but they can't have lots of unusual ingredients that my grocery store doesn't carry. I hate cleaning the kitchen, so I look for easier ways to cook; I've been covered with fresh snow as I stand outside in the winter grilling lamb chops.

If you are still resisting the idea of giving up a little convenience, peek into the dictionary. *Convenience* means "designed for quick and easy preparation or use," but it also means "something conducive to comfort or ease." The latter is the definition of convenience a compassionate carnivore should use. Cooking a meal from humanely raised meat can be a comfort to you and your family—both the act of cooking and the eating itself, and doing this will eventually ease the difficult lives of meat animals.

During the twentieth century, advertisers convinced us that "food conveyed their [women's] affections and fulfillment of duty to their families. In the hands of women, food is love." McDonald's built on this in the 1980s by shifting its marketing emphasis from the product—burgers—and turning instead to marketing "love, a sense of community, and good feelings." In its commercials, McD's called itself "the glue that holds friends and families together . . . reassuring of stability, security, and love."[32]

It's time to take back the idea that fast food is love, that convenience food is stable and secure. Slowing down and cooking for each other is love. Bowling together, slowly, while wearing an apron? That's even better.

# Embracing
# Eggplant

••• ••• •••••• ••• •••

I PAY ATTENTION. I waste less meat. I'm working to replace factory-raised meat with meat from animals raised humanely. But the evidence piles up around me like bones after a barbeque. Since factory farming is bad for the animals and bad for the environment, there is one last step a compassionate carnivore can take.

When sitting in a restaurant, I can be fairly certain the meat is factory-raised, unless the restaurant proclaims otherwise, so I only have two choices—either consume a meal with factory meat and all the externalities that go with it, or consume a meal without meat. These are hard words for this carnivore to type, but if I must choose between factory meat and no meat, I have begun choosing more meatless meals. Besides, by choosing to go meatless instead of consuming factory meat, at the very least I might drop a few pounds so that mypyramid.gov will stop harassing me about my weight.

Choosing a meatless meal over meat from animals raised in a factory feels, in some odd way, un-American, subversive. There's a reason for this. During World War II meat companies made sure homemakers felt it their patriotic duty to feed their men meat. Armour and Company bragged in an ad that "because they were supplying meat and dairy products to the U.S. Army, 'the average soldier gains 7 pounds during his first month in the Army.'"[33] If meat was good for our soldiers, it was good for the people at home, so homemakers, while scrimping in lots of areas during the war, were encouraged to stuff their families full of meat.

The kicker, though, were ads like this put out in the 1950s by the American Meat Institute. Called "Meat and the American Family," the ad showed a "wholesome" family and contained this rousing ad copy: "Since it cut this country out of the wilderness, the American family has always reached for the true, the genuine, and the virile—We were never a bland people—Our wives and mothers plan our meals around flavor—by native preference, the flavor of meat."[34]

I nearly leaped to my feet and saluted when I read that. No wonder meat has become such an integral part of our lives. For most of the twentieth century ads have been pounding this message into the American brain, so it's hard for most of us to step back and think about actively eating less.

But I have successfully begun, now and then, to choose a restaurant meal without the meat. And if all those health advocates are right that too much meat is bad for me, I'll be better off. But I always remember my one rule about changing the way we eat meat, and that's to be compassionate, first, toward yourself. That means that if you're in a restaurant and hate all the meatless options, don't flail yourself with a bamboo cane because you chose the factory meat. If you're exhausted after a day's work and want to be a baby bird being fed by Papa Bird, you're not a bad person. Choosing the meatless meal over factory meat may not amount to a large percentage of your diet, and that's okay, but your choices will be more consistent with your values.

What does it really mean to eat less meat? It means eating more vegetables. For many of you healthy kale–arugula–brussels sprouts lovers out there, this won't be a problem. Some of us, however, have had less than successful relationships with vegetables. We don't know how to cook grain unless it's Minute Rice. Our menu planning and cooking skills have always been centered on meat. It's not that we don't believe you can't survive on less meat, since vegetarians don't seem to be collapsing on the streets around us, it's that change is hard and the idea of replacing meat with something else is intimidating.

Sad to say, I'm not the most creative of cooks. In fact, I can do little without a recipe, and if that recipe has more than seven or eight ingredients to it, I get tired just looking at it. My favorite cookbook is *Desperation Dinners,* an entire book of twenty-minute recipes built on prepackaged foods like soups, frozen veggies, and pasta. The authors are my heroes.

Vegetables and grains have only recently been added to my list of edible foods, so I don't have much experience cooking them. When I realized I needed to reduce my consumption of meat, I decided to have a go at the most frightening of plants, the pleasingly plump and purple eggplant. It didn't go well the first time, and it didn't go well the second time. Soon, all I had to do was say the word "eggplant" to Melissa, and she'd turn a unique shade of purple. A recent book title caught my eye—*Alone in the Kitchen with an Eggplant.* This was intended to be an amusing, comforting book on cooking, but for me, the title called up a Stephen King–like horror novel.

However, I persisted, and because Melissa depends on me to feed her, she continued to bravely show up at the dinner table. Finally, I sliced an eggplant, dipped the slices first in milk, then in loads of crushed garlic (seasoned with a few breadcrumbs), and I fried them. Eureka! Edible eggplant.

I tried falafel, small Middle Eastern fried patties made of ground garbanzo and fava beans. When I had finished struggling with the falafel, nearly in tears, I made us each a peanut butter sandwich. Later I shared my falafel debacle with my friend Pat, who used to be a chef, explaining that the patties soaked up all the oil, fell apart, and then dried into tooth-destroying lumps.

Pat laughed at my pain and said, "Forget making them from scratch. Just buy one of those boxed mixes. They're super easy."

I waited a few beats, then confessed. "That's what I was using."

I have done unspeakable things to rice, but somehow I'm learning, and if I can whip up a few meals without meat, anyone can. I now make a mean steamed broccoli, and have discovered that woman *can* live by quesadillas alone. I've learned that I don't need meat at every meal. A plate without meat is *not* a squadron of soldiers without a leader, or a wheel without a spoke. It's simply a plate of food.

Before I was a farmer, 100 percent of my meat came from a factory. After we started farming and eating our lamb, that figure dropped down to perhaps 90 percent. But since I've been paying attention and working to replace the factory meat, I'm happy to report considerable success. Most weeks, about 50 percent of my meals are made from happy meat, 25 percent are meatless, and 25 percent are from factory meat. It's taken Melissa some time to adjust to the meatless meals. At first, once we moved beyond the eggplant disasters, she'd stare down at the plate, then give me a woeful smile. "No meat, then?"

Some weeks are better than others, of course. In the winter, when our lives slow down, thanks to snow and ice and thirty-below temperatures, I cook more out of our freezer, so the percentage of happy meat rises to 60 or 70 percent. During busier seasons, a week's meals might be one-third humanely raised meat, one-third meatless, and one-third factory meat. Since feeding one's sense of humor is the only way to survive, it does make me chuckle to admit that during the crunch weeks of writing this book, I lacked the energy to cook, and since we couldn't live on Melissa's fried egg sandwiches alone, no matter how delicious they were, Schwan's saved me. We ate nearly 75 percent factory meat meals and 25 percent meatless meals. I accept that there's a gap between my real and ideal and just move on.

Dr. Robert Lawrence of Johns Hopkins University started a movement called "Meatless Monday," which works in part because of the satisfying alliteration. I don't want to be that tied down, so I might practice "Meatless Tuesday Dinner" or "Meatless Friday Lunch" instead.

Talking about eating less meat makes some farmers nervous, but it shouldn't. When *Newsweek* ran ten tips for being "green," and included "Eat your veggies . . . have a meatless Monday," an Iowa farmer responded: "As small-scale cattle farmers, we were not impressed with your idea to save the planet by forgoing meat once or twice a week." Instead, the farmers urged readers to use cloth grocery bags, drive on properly inflated tires, and remove unnecessary items from their trunk.[35]

Being a farmer, the idea that people might start eating less meat doesn't bother me. Perhaps I'll start selling eggplant along with our lamb.

••• ••• •••

Pay attention. Waste less meat. Replace factory meat with humanely raised meat. Go meatless if you can't avoid the factory meat. Each of these steps involves many tiny, seemingly insignificant choices in your week, and when you're focused on the details, it's sometimes hard to see progress. And because the modern meat industry is so massive, a monolith seemingly impervious to change, it's perfectly reasonable to ask one last question: are the actions we're taking making *any* difference?

## Part Eight

# Making a Difference

If you don't like what you're doing, you can always pick
up your needle and move to another groove.

—TIMOTHY LEARY

I've grown accustomed to being different. Whenever I use the word *shepherd* to describe myself, people laugh hysterically, then stop when I don't join them. "You're serious?" they say. "You really call yourself a shepherd?" You think I'd just told them I was a stagecoach driver or a Pony Express rider. People have been herding sheep for ten thousand years, and have been calling themselves that for perhaps as long, so why stop now?

A few years ago I discovered Elvis's blues songs and became an avid Elvis fan. (Melissa might use the word *rabid* instead.) When friends visit my office and are confronted with four Elvis images on the wall, they fall silent, as if they're embarrassed for me. It truly freaks people out that a middle-class, educated, liberal Northerner would not only be an Elvis fan, but would also openly admit it. I continue to be a vocal fan, partly because I love his voice, and partly because it challenges people's stereotypes.

Then of course, there's the whole gay thing. I've known I was gay since I was nineteen, so I've been different for a *very* long time. I've spent my life getting used to being different, then teaching people that although I may be different from them, I'm still a moral, ethical person who has similar wants and needs and fears and dreams.

I like who I am, and while there might be a few other Elvis-loving lesbian shepherds in the country, I'm guessing there aren't many. I'm used to being different.

What does this all have to do with you? Paying attention to where your meat comes from will make you different, especially if you're bowling alone. Eating a vegetarian meal now and then may, in your circles, make you different. Buying meat directly from a farmer instead of from the grocery store will make you different. If you're not used to it, being different can make you feel uncomfortable. It may feel a little weird.

That's okay, because you're living according to your principles. It might just be that the best way to *make* a difference is to *be* different.

# A Seat
# at the Table

... ... ...... ... ...

SOME PEOPLE BELIEVE the best way to help livestock animals is to stop eating them altogether. Yet despite the deeply felt and admirable sentiments behind these calls to vegetarianism, I've always wondered whether the act of becoming a vegetarian or vegan has any positive impact on the lives of animals. Instead, I believe that remaining "at the table," if you will, is more effective than walking away, and as it turns out, the numbers have proved me right.

I picture the whole meat scene as a very long, glossy conference table. Sitting at this table are the big factory farming corporations, the agribusiness companies making convenience and fast food, and the consumers who don't care where their meat comes from, as long as it's inexpensive and readily available and relatively safe to eat. These groups take up most of the table.

But at one end, clutching onto the table for dear life and refusing to be squeezed out entirely, are some "different" people—a small group of sustainable farmers, organic farmers, and small conventional farmers. Crammed in next to us are the compassionate carnivores who are concerned about the animals, the environment, and their own health.

Carnivores speak most loudly not through their words, but by how they spend their food dollars. People who remain at the table and support sustainable, responsible, and humane agriculture by purchasing meat from these farmers are sending a message to those farmers: "Keep doing what you're doing. Don't stop. We'll buy your product."

When consumers purchase our meat, it allows us, the small and sustainable farmers, to remain at the table, to grow and thrive and provide humanely raised meat to increasing numbers of people. Because farming is a business, there won't be a product unless there is a demand.

People who become complete vegetarians for the sake of animals are basically getting up from the table and leaving the room. Although they might work to help better animals' lives through their words, those words won't keep a sustainable farmer in business. Only dollars will. If you don't buy from these farmers, they'll go out of business, and you'll have even fewer choices than you do now. Flexitarians, vegetarians who eat meat occasionally, are remaining at the table. Carnivores who choose to go meatless now and then are remaining at the table.

Twenty years ago, philosophy professor R. G. Frey doubted that vegetarianism would be an effective way to deal with the "painful rearing practices" of commercial farming. Instead, he urged people to identify practices that most disturbed them, and try to convince farmers and agribusiness to address those problems.

Frey recently revisited the issue, and wasn't happy to discover that he'd been right. There are more vegetarians today than ever before. Some estimates put them at 5 percent of the population. It follows that this increase in the number of vegetarians should have resulted in a decrease of meat consumed, but as I discussed earlier, the opposite has occurred. In the last twenty-five years our annual consumption has grown from 177 pounds to 200 per person and is projected to keep growing. As Frey wrote in "Utilitarianism and Moral Vegetarianism Again: Protest or Effectiveness?": "At a time when the very act of becoming a vegetarian was being touted as the 'most effective' step one could take to do something about painful rearing practices, and as more people were taking that step, the number of animals being so reared has skyrocketed to a figure today that is simply gigantic. . . . The entire argument, in short, has been overtaken by the sheer magnitude of increase in the number of animals farmed."[1]

Even the Humane Society recognizes we need to remain at the table: "If the farmer who is giving his pigs the best life he can is not supported by the consumer, then there cannot be any growth in that sector. If everybody who is concerned about inhumane conditions stops eating meat, the farmers who are trying to be humane can't succeed. Support the people who are trying to do the best they can."[2]

Roger Scruton chimes in: "If meat-eating should ever become confined to those who do not care about animal suffering then compassionate farming would cease. . . . All animals would be kept in battery conditions. . . . Where there are conscientious carnivores, however, there is a motive to raise animals kindly."[3]

Since we each need to follow our own path, I wholeheartedly support people's decisions to become vegetarians if that's what they are compelled to do. But if there are carnivores who enjoy eating meat but are considering going veggie for ethical reasons, or vegetarians who'd like to become flexitarians and allow a little meat into their diets but feel too guilty, consider this: the more of us who remain at, or join, the table by seeking out and buying humanely raised meat, the stronger our numbers, and the more animals that will be raised in sustainable, humane systems instead of as widgets in a factory. Those of us voting with our food dollars for better lives for livestock and less damage to the environment can remain at that crowded table, trying to elbow our way in, or we can move to our own table, ignoring the big guys altogether.

Maybe some of the consumers at another table will wonder what all the excitement is about and come join us. Maybe some of the conventional farmers will sit up and take notice. Call me a dreamer, but I have high hopes for small conventional farms. They aren't yet factories, so they haven't committed to that path. It's not too late for a conventional farmer to step back, look at what he or she is doing, and consider making some changes.

My "voices at the table" may seem simplistic, but a farmer can dream, can't she? Besides, there is no denying economic reality— if more people demand meat from animals raised humanely, there will be more farmers raising animals humanely.

*Utne Reader* magazine took a look at this in their January–February 2006 issue. They calculated that if every subscriber to the magazine, which at the time was 225,000 people, made the effort to find one meal a week from meat raised by small, sustainable farmers instead of by factory farms, that shift in revenue would pay the average *annual* income of 3,000 farm families.[4] This is huge.

Even if those same 225,000 people did this just once a month instead of once a week, it would still shift a large share of food income from factories to actual farms.

Stay at the table. If you leave, the animals will have fewer and fewer voices speaking on their behalf. Yes, the animal rights, animal welfare, and environmental groups will keep at it, and they've accomplished much good work through their efforts. But as carnivores, because we're responsible for animals' deaths, we are also responsible for their lives. Paying more attention to where your meat comes from, and making changes in the way you eat meat *does* make a difference.

# Connecting
# the Dots

... ... ...... ... ...

IF MY BORDER collie Robin could run through this book and herd together the four things a carnivore can do, he'd end up with these four ideas:

- Pay attention.
- Waste less meat.
- Replace factory meat with meat from animals raised humanely.
- Choose meatless meals over meat from animals raised in factories.

Following these steps will be like juggling. While some of you may have this skill, most of us don't. You'll drop the ball with one step while focusing on another. Your goals may slip in one area as you succeed in another. Staying focused is really hard. You could post on your refrigerator a photo from a factory farm or an assembly line slaughterhouse, but I'm not sure you would be interested in this sort of jolt every day. Perhaps post a list of what you don't like about raising animals in factories. Or a photo of a happy pig, a happy cow, a happy chicken. For me, this might work better—focusing on the animals as real and alive, living the lives I want them to live.

Focus is hard to maintain when we don't get regular and immediate feedback. When I change my eating habits to lose weight, I get immediate feedback every time I step on the scale. The choice I made yesterday to eat an entire plate of chocolate chip cookies impacts my weight today. If you have stopped smoking, but your kid catches you puffing away out in the garage, crouched down behind the barbeque grill, you'll probably receive immediate feedback on how you're doing with your goal.

I don't receive immediate feedback from my choices to eat more humanely raised meat, much as I won't feel anything different in my day if I make choices to reduce my contribution to global warming, so it's up to me to figure out how to keep my original motivation in mind.

Daily gratitude may help you focus. When I first ate a meal from one of our lambs, I thought I'd be upset, since it'd been so hard to take them to the abattoir. But instead of being sad or upset at the lamb chop on my plate, I was nearly overcome with gratitude. It wasn't the sort of gratitude you feel when someone sacrifices something for you, since the animal I was eating had made no such choice; I'd made the choice for it. But it was a gratitude that came from acknowledging I was eating the flesh of an animal, and in order for me to do that, Melissa and I had worked very hard to be sustainable and humane farmers.

Chef Bill Buford described what happened when he acquired a slaughtered hog in New York City (I'll skip the amusing part where he strapped the two-hundred-pound carcass to the front basket of his Vespa and putted home, then brought the carcass into his building and up the elevator): "We had many meals— four hundred and fifty of them, or what worked out to less than fifty cents a plate—as we ate from the snout . . . to the tail. . . .

But the lesson wasn't in the animal's economy. This pig, we knew precisely, had been slaughtered for our table, and we ended up feeling an affection for it that surprised us."[5]

A woman once e-mailed me with the story of how her farm family dealt with eating their farm animals. When a cow was butchered, the small white packages were labeled with the cow's name, like Raisin. That way, when the family sat down to their roast beef, they knew who to thank in their prayers.

Many carnivores love animals, and we obviously also love meat. When I think about all that goes into the food that keeps me alive, I realize I need to take a moment, every day, to experience gratitude for the farmers who raise animals, for the slaughterhouse workers who kill them, and for the animals themselves.

It is easy to become discouraged and think that factory farming has become such a firmly entrenched part of our food supply that nothing will ever change. Before we get so low that we give up and head for a fast-food restaurant, let's take one more stroll down the columns of the USDA livestock statistics for 2005. But this time, instead of looking at the concentration of animals kept on very large farms and CAFOs (which we've already done), let's just look at the number of farms out there.

Of all the farms finishing cattle and calves, there were 207,000 really big guys with feedlots of one hundred to one thousand head and beyond. How about farmers raising between one and ninety-nine steers? There were 776,000 farms in this category.[6]

That's right. There are nearly four times as many small beef growers as large ones. They have fences. They have barns. They know cattle. Will they be willing to shift to grass, to reducing hormone and antibiotic use? That remains to be seen, but if you are willing to pay more for meat from animals raised humanely, it could happen.

Beef cows are used for breeding, and the farmers then usually sell the calves on the open market to be finished in feedlots. Of the U.S. beef cow operations in 2005, 173,000 farmers had more than fifty head. But there were nearly 600,000 small farms raising between one and forty-nine head. What if some of those operations finished the calves themselves and sold them directly to you for a greater profit than they could make on the open market?

Hogs are really dominated by the big guys, as 26,700 farms held 99 percent of the 2005 hog inventory. But there were 40,000 farms raising between one and ninety-nine hogs. I don't know how to get around the contracts many hog farmers have with the big guys, but wouldn't it be wonderful if some of those 40,000 small hog farmers could finish and sell directly to you?

I know I will sound naive to some, especially some conventional farmers. Sustainable and organic supporters might advise us to forget about the conventional farmer and just focus on the "good guys." But many conventional farmers are good guys.

The small farm is not dead; it's just lost touch with you, the consumer. It is going to take time, money, flexible farmers, and determined carnivores, but we can turn this ship around. Buy small. Buy local. Buy sustainable and organic, urge conventional farmers to get with the program. Watch the transformation begin.

Jim Wallis, author of *The Soul of Politics,* identified signs of transformation that he looks for in the political process to indicate that we are moving away from polarization and toward actually making things happen,[7] and I believe these six signs of transformation can be applied to our meat-eating, meat-purchasing habits:

**Conversion:** We are shifting from not-paying-attention carnivores to more conscious carnivores.

**Compassion:** By admitting we are eating animals, we allow ourselves to feel more compassion for them.

**Community:** We are no longer bowling alone, but are reaching out to others, sharing contacts, sharing freezers, and finding ways to buy meat together.

**Reverence:** Once we acknowledge that our meat used to be an animal, and that the animal has died to feed us, reverence naturally follows.

**Responsibility:** Once we open our eyes and connect the dots between a farmer's barn and the burger on our plate, we know we have a responsibility to improve the lives, and deaths, of livestock animals.

**Imagination:** Once we move away from the easy certainty of both animal rights activists and the spokespeople for industrial agriculture, we can create new ways to connect with farmers, raising animals in new ways and in new places.

Mahatma Gandhi warned us against the seven social sins,[8] but these three really struck me as a compassionate carnivore:

**Commerce without morality.** Selling meat without any thought to whether its creation was a moral act seems wrong. For most animal rights activists, eating meat is immoral. For unconscious carnivores, eating meat has nothing to do with morality. For conscious, compassionate carnivores, *how* the meat is raised is the moral issue.

**Pleasure without conscience.** For years I wolfed down that spiced-pork-chop-on-a-stick without any thought about how that pork chop came to be, or whether my choice to eat that pork chop had a negative effect on the environment, on my health, or on the lives of animals.

**Science without humanity.** Science has given us modern agriculture. It has given us the ability to keep cattle alive long enough to be fed enough grain to reach market weight; given us the ability to pack one hundred thousand chickens in one building and keep them alive long enough to create a profit. It has shown us how to cage hogs and raise them quickly, and how to breed chickens to put on weight quickly rather than observe genetic niceties like performing the mating dance.

I'd like to think humanity means being aware of the impact of our actions, having the capacity to put others first, to make choices based on the good of mankind, not just on our own selfish needs. When I checked my dictionary, I was pleased to find I wasn't that far off. The first definition of *humanity* listed is "the quality or state of being humane."

*Newsweek* recently pointed out the rash of memoirs by people who spent one year *not* doing something, or following strict rules. There was the guy who lived biblically, and the woman who gave up shopping. Another gave up anything made in China, another ate only locally grown food. It is fun to read these accounts, and these books show that, as *Newsweek* wrote, "self-deprivation is strangely hip." Through these "experiments" that impose strict rules and limit choice, the authors "organize the messiness of life," an incredibly appealing idea.[9]

But there's a reason I didn't write *The Year of Eating Only Humanely Raised Meat.* An intense twelve-month period of strict rules and drastic change, while illuminating, is a limited period of self-deprivation that isn't necessarily sustainable. Change that doesn't *last* isn't change; it's a fad.

So instead of hopping on the one-year bandwagon and experimenting with being a compassionate carnivore, make a long-term commitment. Start with "The Half Year of Eating One Meal a Week of Humanely Raised Meat," then work your way up until you reach your goal.

Eating animals raised more humanely isn't a game of temporary self-deprivation. It's an act of respect that will affect the lives of the millions of animals raised and eaten in this country every year. The corporations running the factory farms will not initiate change. The only person who can do that is you.

# Meanwhile,
# Back at the Fair . . .

••• ••• •••••• ••• •••

LAST FALL I once again attended the Minnesota State Fair. I love the fair and the food and the noise and all the silly gadgets people sell using outrageous claims that I nearly fall for every time. This year we stood, rapt, as a man demonstrated a foolproof kit for cutting your own mat boards for framing pictures. No measuring! No math! No worries! Then he mentioned the kit's price and I said, "No way!" Melissa had fallen under the mat board guy's hypnosis and, eyes glazed, was ready to hand over her Visa card until I dragged her beyond his spell-casting range and reminded her we needed that money to buy hay for the animals this winter.

We stood at the DNR's big fishpond, staring down at the lethargic gar, trout, and catfish, and when I looked up, through the trees I saw the sign: Miracle of Birth Center. Funny, when it was in the old building, it was simply the Miracle of Birth barn. Now it was a "Center," evoking an image more science than agriculture.

I decided to visit the center again, since I hadn't asked the questions I'd needed to. This time I remained calm. It wasn't the fair's fault that industrial agriculture puts sows in cages, and in an odd way I was grateful the fair had given me the opportunity to see it for my own eyes.

Same setup as the year before. I examined it more closely and realized I couldn't see the sow's face because she was lying against a solid structure that I recognized as a feed trough. Okay, that's good to know they fed her. An overhead spigot dripped cold water on each sow to help cool her.

This time I found a young woman with long brown hair, narrow black-rimmed glasses, and an intensely helpful smile. I asked how old the piglets were. "One and a half weeks." I asked how often the sow was allowed to stand up. "Oh, they can stand up whenever they want. They just can't turn around." I looked closer and noticed that a few sows had sores matching the location of bolts on the blue steel arms. They could stand, but not easily. I must have looked skeptical. "They don't stand because they're hot and tired," she explained.

Hmmm. "And what about food and water?" I asked.

"They feed the sows after the center closes, because it's noisy." Did she mean the people were too noisy for the sows to eat, or that the sows were too noisy when they ate? I assumed it was the former, since we could barely hear each other over the din of human voices in the center. Rather than interrogating her further, I practiced my Minnesota Nice and let the now slightly defensive young woman go. The details really didn't matter anyway, since I still didn't like the setup. The sow would be confined, unable to walk, turn around, roll on her back, wallow in the mud, or nuzzle her babies for three weeks. Too bad they wouldn't be giving her a Pabst Blue Ribbon to help numb the boredom.

At the end of another long day filled with too much food and too many people, but lots of fun, Melissa went for her malt. I took one last nostalgic walk down Judson Avenue, wistfully stopping near the pork-chop-on-a-stick booth just to inhale the intoxicating cloud hanging above the booth. As I watched people stand in very long lines, I moved closer to the booth and noticed there were little bottles of spice mix for sale.

*¡Caramba!*

That's what made those factory-raised pork chops so tasty in the first place. Surely I could handle putting on my Elvis apron, marinating my own pork chops, and grilling them! I stood in line and bought two bottles of spices for four dollars each.

I was so excited! I was Super-Compassionate Carnivore, able to leap over industrialized meat in awkward hops, inconsistent jumps, occasional stumbles, and unsuccessful acrobatics, but at least I was trying.

The next night, I sprinkled the spices on two pork chops, grilled them, and we sat down at the table to eat. That pork chop tasted just as good as the pork-chop-on-a-stick at the fair.

No, actually, it tasted better.

*Much* better.

# Acknowledgments

This book would not have happened without my editor, Renée Sedliar. Even though she's never raised sheep, she successfully shepherded me through the process of turning my idea into a book.

In addition to Renée, I am so pleased that Wendie Carr, publicity miracle worker, and Matthew Lore, brilliant publisher, made the leap from Marlowe to Da Capo, thereby ensuring my Dream Team remained intact. Who knew authors could be so possessive?

My friends and family were patient as I sequestered myself to meet deadlines. Mom and Jim, and Dad and Bev, graciously visited me when I was too busy to drive to them. Cindy Rogers, Pat Schmatz, Bonnie Graves, Phyllis Root, Ellen Hart, and Lori Lake— thanks for reading drafts, and more importantly, keeping me sane and focused.

I've absorbed so much from the farmers I've met over the years— both sustainable and conventional—and continue to be inspired by their love of hard work, pride in their farms, and respect for their animals. Also, I appreciate all the readers of my memoir, *Hit by a Farm*, who responded to my situation as a "city girl" who'd suddenly come face to face with her meat, by sharing their own farm/meat experiences. While this book isn't the sequel to *Hit by a Farm* that many of you requested, it certainly was inspired by my thirteen years as a farmer. (Besides, since memoir is often about what's gone wrong in one's life, I'm hoping there are no more memoirs in my future.)

Finally, I could not write without the support and encouragement of my partner Melissa. She's been making me laugh every day for twenty-four years.

# Notes

## Part One. What's a Carnivore to Do?

1. James E. McWilliams, "Food That Travels Well," *New York Times,* August 6, 2007, http://www.nytimes.com/2007/08/06/opinion/06mcwilliams.html.

2. Carl Honoré, *In Praise of Slowness: Challenging the Cult of Speed* (New York: HarperCollins, 2004), 278.

3. Jonathan Balcombe, *Pleasurable Kingdom: Animals and the Nature of Feeling Good* (New York: Macmillan, 2006), 210.

4. Nicolette Hahn Niman, "Pig Out," *New York Times,* March 14, 2007, http://www.nytimes.com/2007/03/14/opinion/14niman.html.

5. Nicholas D. Kristof, "Save the Darfur Puppy," *New York Times,* May 10, 2007, http://select.nytimes.com/2007/05/10/opinion/10kristof.html.

6. Samantha Power, *A Problem from Hell: America and the Age of Genocide* (New York: Basic Books, 2002), 505.

7. Paul Slovic, "If I looked at the mass I will never act: Psychic Numbing and Genocide," *Judgement and Decision-Making* 2, no. 2 (April 2007): 87.

8. Danielle Nierenberg, *Happier Meals: Rethinking the Global Meat Industry* (Washington, DC: Worldwatch Institute, 2005), 53.

9. Anthony Browne, "Calf? I Nearly Died," *Guardian* (United Kingdom), April 29, 2001, http://www.guardian.co.uk/footandmouth/story/0,,480158,00.html.

## Part Two. Stuffing Ourselves

1. Nierenberg, *Happier Meals,* 9.

2. Brad Knickerbocker, "Humans' Beef with Livestock: A Warmer Planet," *Christian Science Monitor,* February 20, 2007, http://www.csmonitor.com/2007/0220/p03s01-ussc.html.

3. USDA, www.nass.usda.gov/factbook/tables/ch2table21.jpg.

4. USDA Economic Research Service, "Food Consumption," www.ers.usda.gov/Briefing/Consumption.

5. "United States Leads World Meat Stampede," Worldwatch Institute, July 2, 1998, http://www.worldwatch.org/node/1626.

6. Nierenberg, *Happier Meals,* 11.

7. USDA Economic Research Service, "Agricultural Baseline Projections: Baseline Presentation, 2007–2016," www.ers.usda.gov/Briefing/Baseline/present2007.html.

8. Michael W. Fox, *Eating with Conscience: The Bioethics of Food* (Troutdale, OR: NewSage Press, 1997), 13.

9. The 2006 slaughter figures were 33.8 million cattle, 748,000 calves, 104.8 million hogs, 2.8 million sheep, and 8.9 trillion chickens. In 2006 the U.S. population passed 300 million, a nice round number to use, but since about 5 percent of us are vegetarians, it seems more accurate to use 285 million. Divide the 9,110 million animals slaughtered by 285 million people and you have 32 animals killed per person per year. If we assume an American's average life span is eighty years, that would then be 2,560 animals killed over our lifetime.

10. "FDA's Call for Smaller Restaurant Portions Draws Criticism," *Dallas Morning News,* June 3, 2006. Available at http://health.dailynewscentral.com/content/view/2279/63.

11. Lisa Young and Marion Nestle, "The Contribution of Expanding Portion Sizes to the U.S. Obesity Epidemic," *American Journal of Public Health* 92, no. 2 (February 2002): 246.

12. Matt Wake, "Restaurant Portion Sizes Out of Control," *Upstate Today* (South Carolina), August 16, 2007, http://www.upstatetoday.com/news/2007/aug/16/restaurant-portion-sizes-out-control.

13. Allan Salkin, "Be Yourselves, Girls, Order the Rib-Eye," *New York Times,* August 9, 2007, http://www.nytimes.com/2007/08/09/fashion/09STEAK.html.

14. Brian Bernbaum, "Roast Beef Hogs?" CBS News/The Odd Truth, April 26, 2004, http://www.cbsnews.com/stories/2004/04/27/national/main614053.shtml?source=search_story.

15. Jess Blumberg, "Livin' Large," *Smithsonian,* September 2007, 128.

16. Linda Scott Kantor, et al., "Estimating and Addressing America's Food Losses," USDA Economic Research Service, *Food Review* (Jan.–April 1997): 2–12.

17. Associated Press, "Wasteful Family Kicked out of Iowa Buffet Restaurant," May 5, 2006, http://abclocal.go.com/ktrk/story?section=bizarre&id=4146032.

18. I started with the percentages of consumption of each type of meat given earlier: beef, 36 percent; pork, 27 percent; chicken, 37 percent. Take the amount of meat wasted every day—over 22.5 million pounds—apply those percentages, and you have the pounds of each type of animal thrown away. When an animal is killed, only a certain percentage is edible meat. An 1,100-pound steer may yield around 550 pounds of meat; a 250-pound hog, 165 pounds; a 6-pound chicken, 4 pounds. Use these figures to convert pounds to animals, and you have 15,000 cows, 18,000 hogs, and 2 million chickens.

19. Amy Standen, "Chris Cosentino Doesn't Want to Eat Penis, but If He Has To, He Will," Meatpaper.com, March 2007, www.meatpaper.com/articles/2007/0528_cosentino.html.

## Part Three. Old MacDonald's Farm Is Gone, e-i-e-i-o

1. Winifred Gallagher, *House Thinking: A Room-by-Room Look at How We Live* (New York: HarperCollins, 2006), 16.

2. Kim Severson, "Be It Ever So Homespun, There's Nothing Like Spin," *New York Times,* August 13, 2007, http://www.nytimes.com/2007/01/03/dining/03crun .html?_r=1&oref=login.

3. Thomas Hunt and Charles Burkett, *Farm Animals: Covering the General Field of Animal Industry* (New York: Orange Judd Company, 1920), 29.

4. Shannon Hayes, *The Grassfed Gourmet Cookbook: Healthy Cooking and Good Living with Pasture-Raised Foods* (Hopewell, NJ: Eating Fresh Publications, 2004), 22.

5. Carolyn Dimitri, Anne Effland, and Neilson Conklin, "The 20th Century Transformation of U.S. Agriculture and Farm Policy," USDA Economic Research Service, Economic Information Bulletin Number 3, www.ers.usda.gov/publications/eib3/eib3.pdf.

6. "A History of Modern Agriculture: Farmers and the Land," Agriculture in the Classroom, www.agclassroom.org/gan/timeline/farmers_land.htm.

7. Ken Midkiff, *The Meat You Eat: How Corporate Farming Has Endangered America's Food Supply* (New York: St. Martin's Press, 2004), 2.

8. USDA, *Agriculture Fact Book, 2001–2002* (Washington, DC: USDA), 26, http://www.usda.gov/factbook/2002factbook.pdf.

9. Robert A. Hoppe and David E. Banker, "Structure and Finances of U.S. Farms: 2005 Family Farm Report," Economic Information Bulletin No. EIB–12, May 2006, www.ers.usda.gov/publications/EIB12.

10. Midkiff, *Meat You Eat,* 100.

11. Hunt and Burkett, *Farm Animals,* 491.

12. Midkiff, *Meat You Eat,* 11.

13. Roger Horowitz, *Putting Meat on the American Table: Taste, Technology, Transformation* (Baltimore: Johns Hopkins University Press, 2006), 130.

14. Sherri Brooks Vinton and Ann Clark Espuelas, *The Real Food Revival: Aisle by Aisle, Morsel by Morsel* (New York: Jeremy P. Tarcher, 2005), 48.

15. Peter Singer and Jim Mason, *The Way We Eat: Why Our Food Choices Matter* (New York: Rodale, 2006), 21.

16. Eric Schlosser, *Fast Food Nation: The Dark Side of the All-American Meal* (New York: HarperCollins, 2002), 141.

17. George Pyle, *Raising Less Corn, More Hell: The Case for the Independent Farm and Against Industrial Food* (New York: Public Affairs, 2005), 196.

18. Singer and Mason, *Way We Eat,* 24.

19. Roger Caras, *A Perfect Harmony: The Intertwining Lives of Animals and Humans throughout History* (New York: Simon & Schuster, 1996), 203.

20. Jeff Tietz, "Boss Hog," *Rolling Stone,* December 14, 2006, www.rollingstone.com/politics/story/12840743/porks_dirty_secret_the_nations_top_hog_producer_is_also_one_of_americas_worst_polluters.

21. Hayes, *Grassfed Gourmet,* 134.

22. Linda Riebel and Ken Jacobsen, *Eating to Save the Earth: Food Choices for a Healthy Planet* (Berkeley, CA: Celestial Arts, 2002), 88.

23. Hayes, *Grassfed Gourmet,* 139.

24. Nierenberg, *Happier Meals,* 17.

25. USDA, Statistical Highlights, 2005 and 2006 Tables, "Livestock," http://www.nass.usda.gov/Publications/Statistical_Highlights/2005/tables/livestock.htm and http://www.nass.usda.gov/Publications/Statistical_Highlights/2006/tables/livestock.htm.

26. Michael Pollan, *The Omnivore's Dilemma: A Natural History of Four Meals* (New York: Penguin Press, 2006), 72.

27. Eric Schlosser, *Chew on This: Everything You Don't Want to Know about Fast Food* (Boston: Houghton Mifflin, 2006), 165.

28. Margot Roosevelt, "The Grass-Fed Revolution," *Time,* June 11, 2006, http://www.time.com/time/magazine/article/0,9171,1200759,00.html.

29. Pfizer Animal Health, "Heifer Management Strategies," www.beefheifers.com.

30. Midkiff, *Meat You Eat,* 110.

31. Singer and Mason, *Way We Eat,* 57.

32. Riebel and Jacobsen, *Eating to Save the Earth,* 87.

33. Singer and Mason, *Way We Eat,* 57.

34. Hayes. *Grassfed Gourmet,* 84.

35. Brian DeVore, "Hog Heaven," Summer 2000: Food for Life, *Yes!,* www.yesmagazine.com/article.asp?ID=339.

36. "Think Outside the Crate Campaign," Humane Society of the United States, http://www.hsus.org/farm/camp/totc.

37. Kristian Foden-Vencil, "Kulongoski Signs Ban on Pig Breeding 'Gestation Crates,'" *OPB News,* June 28, 2007, http://www.publicbroadcasting.net/opb/news.newsmain?action=article&ARTICLE_ID=1106103.

38. Andrew Martin, "Burger King Shifts Policy on Animals," *New York Times,* March 28, 2007, http://www.nytimes.com/2007/03/28/business/28burger.html.

39. Alexei Barrionuevo, "Pork Producer Says It Plans to Give Pigs More Room," *New York Times,* January 26, 2007, http://www.nytimes.com/2007/01/26/business/26pigs.html.

40. Tietz, "Boss Hog."

41. Nierenberg, *Happier Meals,* 29.

42. Marika Alena McCauley, "Factory Farms: An Environmental Hazard," Oxfam America,http://www.oxfamamerica.org/whatwedo/where_we_work/united_states /news_publications/food_farm/art2566.html.

43. "Facts about Pollution from Livestock Farms," Natural Resources Defense Council, http://www.nrdc.org/water/pollution/ffarms.asp.

44. Singer and Mason, *Way We Eat,* 65.

45. Nierenberg, *Happier Meals,* 30.

46. Ibid., 32.

47. Singer and Mason, *Way We Eat,* 30.

48. Nierenberg, *Happier Meals,* 30.

49. Singer and Mason, *Way We Eat,* 30.

50. John Roach, "Gulf of Mexico 'Dead Zone' Is Size of New Jersey," *National Geographic News,* May 25, 2005, http://news.nationalgeographic.com/news /2005/05/0525_050525_deadzone.html.

51. Harold Henderson, "Noxious Neighbors," American Planning Association, November 1998, http://www.planning.org/hottopics/hogs.htm.

52. Ibid.

53. Tom Valtin, "I Can Smell for Miles and Miles," *Planet Newsletter,* www .sierraclub.org/planet/200601/tourdestench.asp.

54. Nierenberg, *Happier Meals,* 13.

55. Ibid., 31.

56. Riebel and Jacobsen, *Eating to Save the Earth,* viii.

57. Ibid., xi.

58. Singer and Mason, *Way We Eat,* 31.

59. Associated Press, "Vermont Cows Help Power 330 Homes: Manure-to-Electricity Project Is First to Reach Grid," January 18, 2005, www.msnbc.msn.com /id/6838687.

60. Wade Rawlins, "Hog Farms Try Collecting Gas, Making Energy," *Raleigh News and Observer,* July 29, 2007, www.newsobserver.com/news/story/653245.html.

61. Knickerbocker, "Humans' Beef with Livestock."

62. "Belching Cows: Giant Pills to Counteract the Greenhouse Effect," University of Hohenheim, March 14, 2007, www.bio-pro.de/en/region/stern/magazin/ 03253/index.html.

268 *Notes*

## Part Four. As Green as It Gets

1. Karen Springen, "Fashion: Corn Clothes," *Newsweek,* April 17, 2006, http://www.newsweek.com/id/46045.

2. Michael Pollan, *The Omnivore's Dilemma: A Natural History of Four Meals* (New York: Penguin Press, 2006).

3. Rod Dreher, *Crunchy Cons: The New Conservative Counterculture and Its Return to Roots* (New York: Three Rivers Press, 2006), 68.

4. Vinton and Espuelas, *Real Food Revival,* 169.

5. Anna Kuchment, "What's On Your Label?" *Newsweek* Web Exclusive, March 12, 2007, http://www.newsweek.com/id/36449, and Laura Sayre, "How Do Your Eggs Stack Up?" *Mother Earth News,* April–May 2007, 76.

6. Hayes, *Grassfed Gourmet,* 133.

7. Roger Scruton, "The Conscientious Carnivore," in Steve F. Sapontzis, ed., *Food for Thought: The Debate over Eating Meat* (Amherst, NY: Prometheus Books, 2004), 88.

8. Kim Severson, "Why Roots Matter More," *New York Times,* November 15, 2006,http://www.nytimes.com/2006/11/15/business/smallbusiness/15recall.html?_r=1&ref=smallbusiness&oref=slogin.

9. "The Organic Myth: Pastoral Ideas Getting Trampled as Organic Food Goes Mass Market," *LOHAS Weekly Newsletter,* October 8, 2006, www.lohas.com/articles/83399.html.

10. Quoted in Joseph Hart, "Beyond Organic: Good Food Is about More Than Standards: It's a State of Mind," *Utne Reader,* Jan.–Feb. 2006, 71, http://www.utne.com/2006–01–01/beyond-organic.aspx.

11. "Transitioning to Organic Production," Sustainable Agriculture Research and Education (SARE) SAN/SARE Bulletin, Sustainable Agriculture Network, January 2007, http://www.sare.org/publications/organic/organic.pdf.

12. "Willful Violations," Cornucopia Institute press release, August 31, 2007, Cornucopia Institute, http://cornucopia.org/index.php/willful-violations.

13. Leslie Pave, "Better Meat: An Interview with Niman Ranch's Founder," SustainLane Web site, www.lesliepave.com/pdf/02/better-meat_-an-interview-with-niman-ranchs-founder.pdf.

14. Nina Planck, "Organic and Then Some," *New York Times,* November 23, 2005, http://www.nytimes.com/2005/11/23/opinion/23planck.html?incamp=article_popular.

15. "*Animal Welfare Approved* Standards for Sheep," Animal Welfare Institute, www.awionline.org/farm/standards/sheep.htm.

16. Temple Grandin and Catherine Johnson, *Animals in Translation: Using the Mysteries of Autism to Decode Animal Behavior* (New York: Scribner, 2005), 190.

17. Pollan, *Omnivore's Dilemma,* 79.

18. Jo Robinson, *Pasture Perfect: The Far-Reaching Benefits of Choosing Meat, Eggs, and Dairy Products from Grass-Fed Animals* (Vashon, WA: Vashon Island Press, 2004), 38.

19. Nierenberg, *Happier Meals,* 39.

20. Ibid., 51.

21. Robinson, *Pasture Perfect,* 37.

22. Ibid., 40.

23. Nierenberg, *Happier Meals,* 32.

24. Ibid., 50.

25. Ibid.

26. Cindy Burke, *To Buy or Not to Buy Organic: What You Need to Know to Choose the Healthiest, Safest, Most Earth-Friendly Food* (New York: Marlowe & Co., 2007), 113.

27. Marian Burros, "Chicken with Arsenic? Is That O.K?" *New York Times,* April 5, 2006, http://www.nytimes.com/2006/04/05/dining/05well.html.

28. Hayes, *Grassfed Gourmet,* 14.

29. Ibid.

## Part Five. Choosing How Animals Die

1. American Sheep Industry Association, *Sheep Industry News* 11, no. 1 (January 2007): 16.

2. Richard Bulliet, *Hunters, Herders, and Hamburgers: The Past and Future of Human-Animal Relationships* (New York: Columbia University Press, 2005), 11.

3. "Humane Methods of Livestock Slaughter," Animal Legal and Historical Center, http://www.animallaw.info/statutes/stusfd7usca1901.htm.

4. Kate Roth, "Caring Carnivore," *Yoga Journal,* May 2006, http://www.yogajournal.com/lifestyle/2133.

5. Eric Schlosser, "The Chain Never Stops," *Mother Jones,* July–Aug. 2001, www.motherjones.com/news/feature/2001/07/meatpacking.html.

6. Ibid.

7. Schlosser, *Chew on This,* 179.

8. Dreher, *Crunchy Cons,* 74.

9. "About the HSA," Humane Slaughter Association, http://www.hsa.org.uk/About.htm.

10. Martin, "Burger King Shifts Policy."

11. Grandin and Johnson, *Animals in Translation,* 29.

12. Ibid., 267–68.

13. Ibid., 268.

14. Ibid., 271.

15. *AgMag: Beef,* an agricultural magazine for kids, Illinois Farm Bureau.

16. Hayes, *Grassfed Gourmet,* 18.

17. John Mettler Jr., *Basic Butchering of Livestock and Game* (Pownal, VT: Storey Books, 1986), 6.

18. Scruton, "Conscientious Carnivore," 88.

## Part Six. Time for a Break:
## Taking a Pasture Walk

1. Grandin and Johnson, *Animals in Translation,* 109–10.

2. Cynthia Mills, "Dogs of Rarotonga," June 26, 2004, http://www.discovermagazine.com/2004/jun/dogs-of-rarotonga.

3. Mark Townsend, "Sheep Might Be Dumb, But They're Not Stupid," *The Observer* (United Kingdom), March 6, 2005, http://observer.guardian.co.uk/uk_news/story/0,,1431443,00.html.

4. Singer and Mason, *Way We Eat,* 22.

5. Jonathan Leake, "The Secret Life of Moody Cows," Sunday *Times* Online, February 27, 2005, http://www.timesonline.co.uk/tol/news/uk/article416070.ece.

6. Julianna Kettlewell, "Farm Animals Need 'Emotional TLC,'" BBC News, March 18, 2005, http://news.bbc.co.uk/2/hi/science/nature/4360947.stm.

7. Quoted in Leake, "Secret Life of Moody Cows."

8. Caras, *Perfect Harmony,* 248.

9. Grandin and Johnson, *Animals in Translation,* 55.

10. Ibid., 55–56.

11. Balcombe, *Pleasurable Kingdom,* 221.

12. Ibid.

13. Grandin and Johnson, *Animals in Translation,* 100.

14. Ibid., 69–70.

15. Ibid., 103.

16. Ibid., 104.

17. Richard Bulliet, *Hunters, Herders, and Hamburgers: The Past and Future of Human-Animal Relationships* (New York: Columbia University Press, 2005).

## Part Seven. Bowling Together
## (Slowly, Wearing an Apron)

1. Kim Severson, "Trans Fat Fight Claims Butter as Victim," *New York Times*, March 7, 2007, www.nytimes.com/2007/03/07/dining/07trans.html.

2. Blaire Van Valkenburgh, "The Dog-Eat-Dog World of Carnivores: A Review of Past and Present Carnivore Community Dynamics," in Craig B. Stanford and Henry T. Bunn, eds., *Meat-Eating and Human Evolution* (New York: Oxford University Press, 2001), 116.

3. Robert Putnam, *Bowling Alone: The Collapse and Revival of American Community* (New York: Touchstone, 2001.)

4. Baxter Black, *Horsehoes, Cowsocks, & Duckfeet: More Commentary by NPR's Cowboy Poet and Former Large Animal Veterinarian* (New York: Three Rivers Press, 2002), 142.

5. Putnam, *Bowling Alone,* 22.

6. Neil Genzlinger, "Where Does Your Food Come From?" *Food and Wine,* November 2006, http://www.foodandwine.com/articles/where-does-your-food-come -from.

7. Kim Severson, "Bringing Moos and Oinks into the Food Debate," *New York Times,* July 25, 2007, http://www.nytimes.com/2007/07/25/dining/25sanc.html.

8. Eric Asimov, "In Portland, a Golden Age of Dining and Drinking," *New York Times,* September 26, 2007, http://travel.nytimes.com/2007/09/26/dining/26port .html.

9. Quoted in Hannah Lobel, "Greener Pastures: Ecofriendly strategies for healthier meat-eating," *Utne Reader,* Sept.–Oct. 2007, 80.

10. Christy Harrison, "Rough Cuts," *Plenty*, Aug.–Sept. 2006.

11. Marian Burros, "What the Egg Was First," *New York Times,* February 7, 2007, http://www.nytimes.com/2007/02/07/dining/07eggs.html.

12. Rachel Hutton, "Pecks and the City," *Minnesota Monthly,* March 2007, 64, http://www.minnesotamonthly.com/media/Minnesota-Monthly/March–2007 /Pecks-and-the-City.

13. Laura Sayre, "How Do Your Eggs Stack Up?" *Mother Earth News,* April–May 2007, 72, http://www.motherearthnews.com/Whole-Foods-and-Cooking/2007 –04–01/How-Do-Your-Eggs-Stack-Up.aspx.

14. Catherine Price, "A Chicken on Every Plot, a Coop in Every Backyard," *New York Times,* September 19, 2007, http://www.nytimes.com/2007/09/19 /dining/19yard.html?_r=1&oref=slogin.

15. Margot Roosevelt, "The Grass-fed Revolution," *Time,* June 12, 2006, http://www.time.com/time/magazine/article/0,9171,1200759,00.html.

16. Kim Severson, "Suddenly, the Hunt Is On for Cage-Free Eggs," *New York Times,* August 12, 2007, http://www.nytimes.com/2007/08/12/us/12eggs.html?_r=2&oref =slogin&oref=slogin.

17. Ibid.

18. "Structural and Financial Characteristics of US Farms," 2001 Family Farm Report, USDA Economic Research Service Ag Information Bulletin, #AIB768, May 2001, 70.

19. Dreher, *Crunchy Cons,* 177.

20. Quoted in Dreher, *Crunchy Cons,* 84.

21. Gallagher, *House Thinking,* 85.

22. Schlosser, *Chew on This,* 104.

23. Vinton and Espuelas, *Real Food Revival,* 188.

24. Katherine J. Parkin, *Food Is Love: Food Advertising and Gender Roles in Modern America* (Philadelphia: University of Pennsylvania Press, 2006), 3.

25. Ibid., 95.

26. Andrew Kimbrell, ed., *The Fatal Harvest Reader: The Tragedy of Industrial Agriculture* (Sausalito, CA: Foundation for Deep Ecology, 2002), 285.

27. Vinton and Espuelas, *Real Food Revival,* 187.

28. Marc David, "The Pleasure Principle," *Utne Reader,* Nov.–Dec. 2005, 96.

29. Martin J. Smith and Patrick Kiger, *Poplorica: A Popular History of the Fads, Mavericks, Inventions, and Lore That Shaped Modern America* (New York: HarperCollins, 2004), 120.

30. Ibid., 126.

31. Slow Food brochure, www.slowfoodusa.org.

32. Parkin, *Food Is Love,* 34.

33. Ibid., 95.

34. Ibid.

35. Joan Raymond, "Easy to Be Green," *Newsweek,* January 8, 2007, http://www .newsweek.com/id/56722.

## Part Eight. Making a Difference

1. R. G. Frey, "Utilitarianism and Moral Vegetarianism Again: Protest or Effectiveness?" in Sapontzis, *Food for Thought,* 120.

2. Dennis Rodkin, "Vegetarianism vs. Mindful Meat Eating," *Conscious Choices,* November 7, 2002, http://www.consciouschoice.com/2002/cc1511/vegvsmeat1511 .html.

3. Roger Scruton, "Eating our Friends," Right Reason blog, May 25, 2006, http:// rightreason.ektopos.com/archives/2006/05.

4. Hart, "Beyond Organic."

5. Bill Buford, "Carnal Knowledge: How I Became a Tuscan Butcher," Notes of a Gastronome, *New Yorker,* May 1, 2006, 47, http://www.newyorker.com/archive /2006/05/01/060501fa_fact.

6. USDA, Statistical Highlights, 2006 Tables, "Livestock," http://www .nass.usda.gov/Publications/Statistical_Highlights/2006/tables/livestock.htm.

7. Jim Wallis, *The Soul of Politics: A Practical and Prophetic Vision for Change* (New York: New Press, 1994), 147.

8. "Seven Social Sins," Mani Bhavan Web site, http://www.gandhi-manibhavan .org/main/q7.htm.

9. Jennie Yabroff, "A Year of Selling Books," *Newsweek*, October 1, 2007, 84.

# Resources

## Books for Further Reading

Balcombe, Jonathan. *Pleasurable Kingdom: Animals and the Nature of Feeling Good.* New York: Macmillan, 2006.

Bulliet, Richard W. *Hunters, Herders, and Hamburgers: The Past and Future of Human-Animal Relationships.* New York: Columbia University Press, 2005.

Burke, Cindy. *To Buy or Not to Buy Organic: What You Need to Know to Choose the Healthiest, Safest, Most Earth-Friendly Food,* New York: Marlowe & Co., 2007.

Caras, Roger A. *A Perfect Harmony: The Intertwining Lives of Animals and Humans throughout History.* New York: Simon & Schuster, 1996.

Dreher, Rod. *Crunchy Cons: The New Conservative Counterculture and Its Return to Roots.* New York: Three Rivers Press, 2006.

Fox, Michael W. *Eating with Conscience: The Bioethics of Food.* Troutdale, OR: NewSage Press, 1997.

Gallagher, Winifred. *House Thinking: A Room-by-Room Look at How We Live.* New York: HarperCollins, 2006.

Grandin, Temple, and Catherine Johnson. *Animals in Translation: Using the Mysteries of Autism to Decode Animal Behavior.* New York: Scribner, 2005.

Grew, Raymond, ed. *Food in Global History.* Boulder, CO: Westview Press, 1999.

Hayes, Shannon. *The Grassfed Gourmet Cookbook: Healthy Cooking and Good Living with Pasture-Raised Foods.* Hopewell, NJ: Eating Fresh Publications, 2004.

Honoré, Carl. *In Praise of Slowness: How a Worldwide Movement Is Challenging the Cult of Speed.* New York: HarperCollins, 2004.

Horowitz, Roger. *Putting Meat on the American Table: Taste, Technology, Transformation.* Baltimore: Johns Hopkins University Press, 2006.

Hunt, Thomas, and Charles Burkett. *Farm Animals: Covering the General Field of Animal Industry.* New York: Orange Judd Company, 1920.

Kimbrell, Andrew, ed. *The Fatal Harvest Reader: The Tragedy of Industrial Agriculture.* Sausalito, CA: Foundation for Deep Ecology, 2002.

Midkiff, Ken. *The Meat You Eat: How Corporate Farming Has Endangered America's Food Supply.* New York: St. Martin's Press, 2004.

Montgomery, Sy. *The Good, Good Pig: The Extraordinary Life of Christopher Hogwood.* New York: Ballantine Books, 2006.

Nierenberg, Danielle. *Happier Meals: Rethinking the Global Meat Industry.* Washington, DC: Worldwatch Institute, 2005.

Parkin, Katherine J. *Food Is Love: Food Advertising and Gender Roles in Modern America.* Philadelphia: University of Pennsylvania Press, 2006.

Pollan, Michael, *The Omnivore's Dilemma: A Natural History of Four Meals*. New York: Penguin Press, 2006.

Putnam, Robert D. *Bowling Alone: The Collapse and Revival of American Community*. New York: Touchstone, 2001.

Pyle, George. *Raising Less Corn, More Hell: The Case for the Independent Farm and Against Industrial Food*. New York: Public Affairs, 2005.

Riebel, Linda, and Ken Jacobsen. *Eating to Save the Earth: Food Choices for a Healthy Planet*. Berkeley, CA: Celestial Arts, 2002.

Robinson, Jo. *Pasture Perfect: The Far-Reaching Benefits of Choosing Meat, Eggs, and Dairy Products from Grass-Fed Animals*. Vashon, WA: Vashon Island Press, 2004.

Sapontzis, Steve F., ed. *Food for Thought: The Debate over Eating Meat*. Amherst, NY: Prometheus Books, 2004.

Schlosser, Eric. *Chew on This: Everything You Don't Want to Know about Fast Food*. Boston: Houghton Mifflin, 2006.

———. *Fast Food Nation: The Dark Side of the All-American Meal*. New York: HarperCollins, 2002.

Singer, Peter, and Jim Mason. *The Way We Eat: Why Our Food Choices Matter*. New York: Rodale Press, 2006.

Smith, Martin J., and Patrick Kiger. *Poplorica: A Popular History of the Fads, Mavericks, Inventions, and Lore That Shaped Modern America*. New York: HarperCollins, 2004.

Stanford, Craig B., and Henry T. Bunn, eds. *Meat-Eating and Human Evolution*. New York: Oxford University Press, 2001.

Vinton, Sherri Brooks, and Ann Clark Espuelas. *The Real Food Revival: Aisle by Aisle, Morsel by Morsel*. New York: Jeremy P. Tarcher, 2005.

Wallis, Jim. *The Soul of Politics: A Practical and Prophetic Vision for Change*. New York: New Press, 1994.

## Organizations and Web Sites for Finding Farmers
State or Regional Sustainable Farming Associations or Networks

Remember that most of these organizations were begun as a way for farmers to share information and offer one another support. Some have found ways to reach out and connect consumers with farmers, while others haven't gotten that far in the process.

**Alabama Sustainable
Agriculture Network**
P.O. Box 18782
Huntsville, AL 35804
(256) 751-3925
http://www.asanonline.org

**Appalachian Sustainable
Agriculture Project**
729 Haywood Road
Asheville, NC 28806
(828) 236-1282
http://www.asapconnections.org

**California Certified Organic
Farmers (CCOF)**
2155 Delaware Avenue, Suite 150
Santa Cruz, CA 95060
(831) 423-2263
http://ccof.org

**The Carolina Farm
Stewardship Association**
P.O. Box 448
Pittsboro, NC 27312
(919) 542-2402
http://carolinafarmstewards.org

**Community Involved in
Sustaining Agriculture**
1 Sugarloaf Street
South Deerfield, MA 01373
(413) 665-7100
http://www.buylocalfood.com

**Future Harvest**
(Chesapeake Alliance for Sustainable
Agriculture)
P.O. Box 1544
Eldersburg, MD 21784
(410) 549-7878
http://www.futureharvestcasa.org

**Innovative Farmers of Ohio**
5555 Airport Highway, Suite 100
Toledo, OH 43615
(800) 372-6092
http://firegod.com/xoops/html/
modules/smartsection

**The Kerr Center for
Sustainable Agriculture**
P.O. Box 588
Poteau, OK 74953
(918) 647-9123
http://kerrcenter.com

**Maine Organic Farmers
and Gardeners Association**
P.O. Box 170
294 Crosby Brook Road
Unity, ME 04988
(207) 568-4142
http://mofga.org

**Michigan Agricultural Stewardship
Association (MASA)**
605 N. Birch Street
Kalkaska, MI. 49646
(231) 258-3305

**Nebraska Sustainable
Agriculture Society**
Executive Director: Elaine Cranford
P.O. Box 84764
Lincoln, NE 68501-4764
(402) 770-1705
http://nebsusag.org

**Northeast Organic Farming
Association (NOFA)**
(Chapters in CT, MA, NH, NJ,
NY, RI, VT)
http://www.nofa.org

**Northern Plains Sustainable
Agriculture Society**
P.O. Box 194
LaMoure, ND 58458
(701) 883-4303
(Members mostly in ND, SD, MN,
MT, IA, WY, NB)
http://www.npsas.org

**Ohio Ecological Food and
Farm Association**
P.O. Box 82234
Columbus, OH 43202
(614) 421-2022
http://oeffa.org

**Organic Valley Family
of Farms**
CROPP Cooperative
One Organic Way
LaFarge, WI 54639
(888) 444-6455
http://organicvalley.coop

**Pennsylvania Association for
Sustainable Agriculture (PASA)**
114 West Main Street
P.O. Box 419
Millheim, PA 16854
(814) 349-9856
http://pasafarming.org

**Practical Farmers of Iowa**
P.O. Box 349
Ames, IA 50010
(515) 232-5661
http://practicalfarmers.org

**Rural Roots, Inc.**
(ID, eastern WA, and eastern OR)
P.O. Box 8925
Moscow, ID 83843
(208) 883-3462
http://www.ruralroots.org

**Sustainable Farming
Association of MN**
29731 302 Street
Starbuck, MN 56381
(866) 760-8732
http://www.sfa-mn.org/index.php

**Texas Organic Farmers
and Gardeners Association**
(See Web site for contact information
for your region)
http://tofga.org

## Other Organizations That Might Be Helpful

**American Grassfed Association**
(Site includes a list of producers
who raise animals on grass.)
1648 Gaylord Street
Denver, CO 80206
(877) 774-7277
http://americangrassfed.org

**American Pastured Poultry
Producers Association**
(Site features a producer directory,
letting consumers search for farmers
by state.)
36475 Norton Creek Road
Blodgett, OR 97326
(541) 453-4557
http://apppa.org

**California Coalition for
Food and Farming**
406 Main Street, #313
Watsonville, CA 95076
(831) 763-2111
http://www.calfoodandfarming.org

**Cascade Harvest Coalition**
4649 Sunnyside Avenue North,
Room 123
Seattle, WA 98103
(206) 632-0606
http://cascadeharvest.org

**Chefs Collaborative**
(Partners in local, artisanal,
sustainable cuisine)
89 South Street, Lower Level
Boston, MA 02111
(617) 236-5200
http://chefscollaborative.org

**Community Alliance with
Family Farmers**
36355 Russell Boulevard
P.O. Box 363
Davis, CA 95617
(530) 756-8518
http://www.caff.org

**Earth Pledge Farm to Table**
("Earth Pledge is a nonprofit organization that promotes sustainable develop-
ment by identifying and implementing
innovative technologies that balance
human and natural systems.")
http://farmtotable.org

**Eat Well Guide**

(Enter your zip code, the number of miles you're willing to travel, and the site finds the farmers, stores, and restaurants near you that offer sustainable food.)

215 Lexington Avenue, Suite 1001
New York, NY 10016
(212) 991-1858
http://eatwellguide.org

**Farmers Markets**

(Click on your state for a list of farmers markets.)
http://www.ams.usda.gov/farmersmarkets

**Food Routes Network**

(This site's "Find Good Food" map helps you locate farmers, farmers markets, restaurants, food coops, and CSAs near you.)

P.O. Box 55
35 Apple Lane
Arnot, PA 16911
(570) 638-3608
http://foodroutes.org
(Similar information can be accessed through http://www.localharvest.org.)

**Meatless Monday**

(In association with the Johns Hopkins Bloomberg Public School of Health, site provides health and nutrition information, recipes, and encouragement for going without meat one day a week.)

**Meatless Monday Campaign, Inc.**

215 Lexington Avenue, Suite 1001
New York, NY 10016
http://www.meatlessmonday.com

**Midwest Organic and Sustainable Education Service**

P.O. Box 339
Spring Valley, WI 54767
(715) 772-3153
http://mosesorganic.org

# Index